All Shook Up

My Natural Fight Against Cancer
(with a little help from Elvis)

by Suzie Derrett
as told to Juliet Sullivan

Magic Waters

Gary & Suzie Derrett
604.541.0018
svderrett@hotmail.com
www.suziedyourbodyiswater.com

Thank you to the following authors for allowing us to re-publish their quotes:

Alan Cohen: *"A Deep Breath of Life,"* published by
Hay House Publishing
www.AlanCohen.com

Robert Wright: *"Killing Cancer - Not People"*
American Anti-Cancer Institute
www.americanaci.org

Marianne Williamson: *"Illuminata,"* published by Random House
www.marianne.com

Susan D'Agostino: *"Hello Susan, it's me – cancer"*
www.healingeverybody.com

TABLE OF CONTENTS

A NOTE FROM THE WRITER:

When Suzie asked me to write her book, I did not hesitate. Hers is a story that needs to be told, and I am honoured to be the one she has chosen to tell it. I met Suzie through her daughter Shannon, one of my dearest friends. When Shannon was diagnosed with breast cancer at age 40, I was shocked and saddened, and so began my own journey – of learning and discovery.

I had never before experienced the impact of cancer on someone close to me. I knew nothing of the disease itself, the treatment, the alternatives, or its devastating effects.

It was incomprehensible to me that my friend Shannon – just 40, beautiful, fit, the picture of vitality, and a health enthusiast – would be going through this. But she was. When I received the first phone call – to tell me yes, it was a cancerous lump – I cried. I cried on the phone with Shannon, and later, I cried alone. It took me a long time to accept it.

I quickly learned about all of those things that I had previously been blissfully unaware of. I learned about tumours and biopsies and lumpectomies and mastectomies. I was there at the hospital when Shannon went for her mastectomy, and I cried with her when they took her away for the operation, hand held high in salute to the battle ahead. If it felt like a hazy, surreal nightmare to me, I cannot imagine how it felt to her.

I watched Suzie cry as her daughter was wheeled away, but she seemed so composed and resolute, that I also felt calmed and un-afraid. The fear I had felt in the first days of the diagnosis and the following tests, strangely disappeared that day. Suzie never had a doubt that Shannon would beat this thing, and so neither did I.

One Sunday morning, sometime after the mastectomy, I was summoned to a meeting at Shannon and her husband Steve's house, along with two other good friends and both families, to watch a film about The Gerson and to learn what my friend's life would entail over the next few months. This is the treatment that Shannon had chosen, and this is how we would learn about it. To me, it was daunting, and terrifying; an unknown concept, and one that I did not fully understand. But I did not question it. She was determined, and I believe that no-one has the right to question a determination that is such a personal choice. I decided that I would just be there, to support, if needed; not to judge, question, or con-demn.

But I cannot lie; I was worried, and confused. What the hell was a coffee enema? This was so completely opposite to what we are brought up to believe in; we are taught to believe in doctors, medicine, conventional, scientific treatments; especially when it comes to something as big and nasty as cancer. I had not read the books that Shannon had; I had not had the experience Suzie had.

Over the next few months, I watched my friend go through a tough and terrible time, as she withdrew from a normal life and concentrated on one of pure survival. Her days were full of juicing, enemas, injections, vitamins and sleep. She was exhausted, thin and scared. I, on the other hand, was just scared.

Through all of this, Suzie's unwavering faith in Shannon's re-covery was awe-inspiring. And I began to develop a little of that faith. As Shannon's tumour markers dropped, and her health and vitality came back, I began to relax. I began to believe.

Shannon is back to living a normal life now, not one in fear or darkness, but one of hope and survival; just like her Mom. These are two amazingly determined women, and I am in awe of their bravery, faith and strength.

I didn't know Suzie as she was going through her cancer battles, but through writing this book, I have come to know her, and her story, well. And what a story it is.

Thank you, Suzie, for giving me the opportunity to tell it.

—Juliet Sullivan

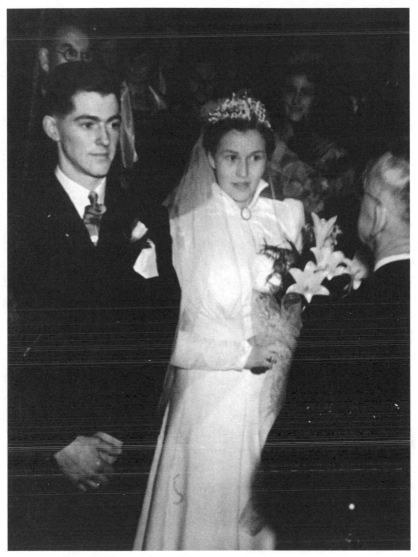

My parents

This book is dedicated to
my wonderful parents who gave me life,
and taught me that *"This too shall pass"*.

Suzie Derrett

FOREWORD

BY

DR UDO ERASMUS

We love stories in which someone wins against all odds. This is one such story. In fact, it is a story of three people who bucked the system, and all of them won. It is a story of pain and fear, of anger and resolve, of love, and of fierce determination.

The Derrett story of beating cancer with a little help from friends—like Charlotte Gerson, Mother Nature, and old, stale, dirty (tap) water made fresh again—can inspire and bring hope to many people.

I witnessed a part of that story. A mutual friend had invited me to the Derrett residence, to see if I could help Suzie's husband Gary with my knowledge of health. It's what I do for a living. At that time, I was working with healthy oils. I had written a book entitled *"FATS THAT HEAL FATS THAT KILL,"* had developed methods for making oils with health in mind, had used that method to intro-duce flax oil to the world, and had moved on to Udo's Oil, a better balanced blend of oils containing all that's good in the arena of fats, and free of all that's bad. Many people have used it to improve their health. When I went to see Gary, I thought that he would be no exception.

Gary was sitting in the left corner of his couch. He calls himself 'Dead Man Walking' in the book. I saw him as 'Dead Man Sitting'; pale and motionless. Worse, he appeared to be completely uninterested in life.

Very quickly, I realised that he was beyond my help. I remember talking to him about peace, because I knew he was headed there—you know, the peace AFTER life—so I thought I could best serve him by being calm and focusing on acceptance of the inevitable.

I went home upset. I hate it when I cannot help people. The end of Gary, I figured, and got on with my life.

About a year and a half later, I met a completely different Gary. His cheeks were pink. He was animated, charged, and active. His health and energy had been completely restored. He credits his wife Suzie with engineering his recovery.

If chemo, radiation, or surgery did NOT restore his health and energy, then what did?

Gary and 'his women' are proof that we do not need to poison our way to health. In fact, health comes from taking steps to live more in line with the forces that designed health on planet Earth: life and nature.

But let me stop here. I can give you the theory. The Derrett family is living proof of its practical application. I love the feistiness of their attitude in the face of the terminal diagnosis. And especially, I love the three happy endings!

Enjoy their story.

Dr Udo Erasmus
www.udoerasmus.com

Introduction

"There is no more important message to learn and teach your loved ones than... only you can heal yourself."

—*Robert G Wright*

You could say that I am an Elvis Presley fan. Even now, 56 years after I first heard his voice, and 35 years after he died, his songs can bring me to tears – both of joy and sadness. I still listen to his songs every single day. In fact, when I am in my car alone, I *only* listen to Elvis.

My connection to Elvis goes back to when I was 11 years old and I first heard him on the radio. His voice captivated me, before I ever saw his face.

I remember clearly the first time I ever saw him on TV. He was on the Ed Sullivan show, and there had been a two week build-up to the event, with my Dad teasing me for that whole time about my eagerness and anticipation. On the night of the show, Dad made popcorn and we sat down to watch, Dad mildly amused and me wildly excited. It was 1956. I remember being transfixed, and the world suddenly became a richer, deeper place, full of wonder. I was mesmerised by his magic; his charisma, and although of course I wasn't aware of his impact as a young girl, I now realise that I was moved in a deep, profound way that has never left me.

I never wanted to be his girlfriend or wife, though - like most of the female population at the time. I wanted to be his sister. I wanted to share my world with him, and in some remote way, I feel that I have done just that. I feel that Elvis has accompanied me through my journey of life.

Fast forward 20 years, to one balmy evening in June 1977, when I was a young mother of four... I was curled up on the couch at home, excited to watch what I had no idea would be Elvis' last televised concert. My girls were all busy and Gary, my husband, was in his workshop. I had been impatiently waiting for 'The King's' arrival on the screen, counting down the minutes until his performance. When he finally came on stage, he looked shockingly bloated and unhealthy, and I was so shaken by his change in appearance that I let out a guttural scream that brought my husband Gary running in from outside, thinking something had happened to one of our daughters.

Elvis died six weeks later, and on that dark, miserable day, I received calls from all over the world from people who knew me, to ask if I was OK. Like I had lost a brother. I wasn't OK, of course. I was deeply affected by his death, more so that I could have imagined. In fact, every day for a year after Elvis died, the radio station CJOR played *My Way*, and every day for a year, I listened to that song, and cried. That was the strength of my connection to Elvis, and even now, long after his death, I still feel it.

Elvis, I believe, has helped me cope with, overcome, and soothe the trauma in my life – and there has been lots.

I have been carrying the premise of this book around in my head for many years. Those close to me, and many people I have met throughout my journey, when told about the concept, have questioned why I have not yet written it.

The fact is, it's not easy to write a book; especially one that lays bare the soul, delves into the deep, dark corners of life, and one that challenges popular belief. So for years, I put it off to one side, where it niggled at me daily, and woke me in the night.

And then, in May of 2012, on my 67th birthday, at my friend Sharon's 65th birthday party, I met two people who inspired me to sit down and finally do it.

Sharon's daughter Sage is married to Anthony Robbins, and that night, Sage and Tony had arranged a big surprise birthday party for Sharon. Knowing how much Sharon loves Elvis, they had flown in Shawn Klush, the brilliant Elvis impersonator, to sing at the birthday party.

One of Shawn's Sweet Inspirations back-up singers was an original Elvis back-up singer. You can imagine how excited I was to watch her perform alongside Shawn, and later I tracked her down to speak to her. I told her about my Elvis obsession, though I may not have called it an obsession. I then told her about my idea for this book. She grasped me excitedly by the shoulders, looked deep into my eyes, and said in her heavy Southern drawl, "Girl – you have to write this book." Something in her eyes, and her vice-like grasp on my shoulders, spoke to me.

The other person I talked to that night was Tony Robbins. When I finally got to speak to him (Tony is always popular at a party), I related the story of my chat with the back-up singer earlier in the evening. Tony asked what the book was going to be about. I told him that it was my account of my battles with cancer, and how I wanted to share with the world my own experience of how I beat it – twice – naturally – without ever taking any drugs. He grasped both my shoulders, looked deep into my eyes, and said "Girl – you have to write this book!" He may not have grasped my shoulders, but he did tell me I must write this book. When you are told by the great Anthony Robbins that you should write a book, you go away and do it. So here I am, doing it.

This is my story, and it has been a long, tumultuous, sometimes terrifying, journey. I was diagnosed with breast cancer at age 52, and uterine cancer at age 60. I survived. As well as husband Gary, I believe that Elvis got me through it. Hence the title of this book, and all of its chapters; all songs recorded by Elvis. By giving these chapters in this book and my life these song titles, I am dedicating them to the (second) hero and constant companion in my life (Gary didn't ever record any songs, so Elvis was the natural choice).

All Shook Up is written solely to bring hope to all those going through a similar struggle in their lives. It is not an instruction manual, a medical journal, or a how-to guide. It not a moral judgement. It is not intended to preach, lecture or advocate. It is intended simply to tell the story of how I fought and beat cancer – twice – without chemo, radiation or conventional medicine. My way.

CHAPTER ONE
HARD HEADED WOMAN

"Cancer is a word, not a sentence."

—John Diamond

July 1997 – Surrey, BC, Canada

It had been a beautiful, happy day. I was lying on a sun lounger by our swimming pool, husband Gary beside me, drinking iced tea in the late afternoon sun. It was our 32nd wedding anniversary and we were surrounded by family. Our four grown-up daughters were laughing and chatting as they watched their children, our grandchildren, splashing in the pool. The sun was setting in the distance, and I was filled with a sense of calm and happiness.

It was a perfect moment, but it changed suddenly into a terrible one, instantly and without preamble.

My 2 year old grandson Triston had climbed onto my lap so we could look up at the darkening sky. He pointed up at something and accidentally hit my breast with his elbow. It was immediately painful; more than it should have been for a simple knock. My hand went instinctively to my breast, and there, I found a lump.

Intuition is a powerful indicator, and I believe we have a connection to our bodies that doesn't often lie. In this case I would have been happy to have been wrong, but I just had this deep, knowing instinct. I had some experience of breast cancer too - my mother had fought it some years earlier - and as I sat there in the sun, hand glued to my breast, I just *knew* that something wasn't right.

Pushing the sick feeling of dread to the back of my mind, I carried on with the family party. Family is everything to me, and watching my grandchildren having fun was more important than the worry that I felt, and the fear I knew I would soon have to deal with.

The next day, I went to my doctor, a doctor I had come to know well, and trust. He examined me and said sternly, "Because of your family history, I am sending you for a mammogram, right now."

Right now? I mean, I am all for a quick diagnosis – but right now? Things were going so fast. But I did what I was told. The doctor and I were almost friends and I knew he was pulling strings for me. So I went.

When they did the mammogram, I felt something pop. People will tell you that can't happen, but I have discovered since – yes it can. It did. Something changed that day. I firmly believe that the mammogram released the cancer cells into my body.

My doctor arranged for me to have a biopsy that same day. Again, things were moving quickly, and I wasn't given much time to think.

As I was lying on the table having the biopsy, the doctor said to me, "So, Suzie, what would you do if you found out this was breast cancer?" I didn't need to think too hard about that one. Without further explanation, I calmly said, "Oh I know what I'd do." I was casual, but resolute.

A few days later, I got the call. I had been with the family at a work event in Vancouver. Gary and I owned a few vacuum cleaner stores, and we had been in Vancouver at a demonstration given by one of the manufacturers. When we walked in the door of our home, after a long, tiring day, the phone was ringing. I answered the call with trepidation. My doctor said to me, "Suzie, I've got some bad news for you." I don't remember anything else. You hear those words, and everything changes. You've got it. The best way I can describe the impact is – I was *all shook up*. It's a perfect description of the swirl of emotions, the confusion, the absolute blanket of fear that descended upon me.

Despite the all-consuming terror, I put it out of my head. I was surrounded by people and I wasn't going to let them see me upset. Also, my daughter Lori was visiting from Seattle and staying with us in the house, so I didn't have time to deal with anything else. I told no-one about the phone call. I went to bed that night and, strangely enough, I slept really well. Gary did too – none the wiser that his wife had been diagnosed with cancer. When I did tell him the next day, he was surprisingly calm – like he knew that I could beat it. He knew his wife was a fighter.

That next morning, I drove over to my girlfriend Vicky's house. She lived on the river and I always found her house to be something of a sanctuary. I said to her, "I just need a place to lie down and think for a while." I did just that. I went to sleep, I meditated, I reflected. We chatted. Slowly, I got my head around it. What came to me that day was this: Out of this experience, what is the very worst thing that can happen to me? I could die. So I am going to give this all I've got, and I am going to *live* until I die. And I am not going to let the fear get me. You have to work on it, and it's tough, but I knew that I would still sleep at night. I would still live my life.

When I got my pathology report, it turned out that I had had the lump for 12 and a half years. I had never found it, Gary had never found it, mammograms had never found it. I had been oblivious to this thing which had been living in my body for over 12 years.

After the day that my grandson Triston accidentally hit me, it was sore, and the soreness wouldn't go away. There was a push from the doctors to get the tumour out right away. But I had had it, lived with it, and never been affected by it, for 12 and a half years. It was hard to digest.

But I knew something changed when I had the mammogram, and it just didn't feel right. I just felt that the cancer cells had been released into my body. I knew I needed to use my brain and get it out. So I had a mastectomy as soon as I could.

The night before the surgery, I took my girls out for dinner and gave them each a book on being strong. I had been through this with my own mother, and I knew it was a tough experience for them to go through. My mum had had a radical mastectomy but she had beaten it. At dinner, my girls were surprisingly calm. I think it might be because I didn't make a big deal out of it, and because they knew I was strong.

I was strong because I had to be. Cancer is an isolating, insular and very personal disease. You are fighting against something in your own body. It's you versus the cancer. It has no feelings, it has no shame. I became a one woman warrior, determined and bold. I had to be.

The next morning, Gary dropped me off, and I walked into the hospital alone. Like most people, I dislike being in a hospital – I just want to get in and get out as fast as I can - and that day, I didn't want anybody there. I had all my Elvis CDs with me, and I was scheduled for the operation at 10am. They finally took me at 2pm. I was waiting, listening to my music, trying to still my racing mind. I remember looking over at the nurses, and someone asking the orderly what he'd given to calm me. He said, "She doesn't want anything - she has Elvis."

He let me listen to Elvis all the way up to the operating room.

When I awoke, I had one less breast and 17 less lymph nodes. They had taken the lymph nodes from my right arm. After testing, cancer was found to be in just one of them.

In retrospect, I would not have allowed them to take the lymph nodes. But it was all so rushed and then I didn't know any different. My arm has never recovered from that; it was just too drastic. I was bitten by a mosquito once on that arm a few years ago and it doubled in size. I can't have blood taken from that side, and I can't have my Vitamin C drips on that arm. (Vitamin C drips became a regular part of my life, and still are to this day.) I have to be really careful now with that arm.

It was scary because with my mom they had taken twice as many lymph nodes as they did with me, and her arm never recovered; in fact it was double the size of mine. She had to wear a tensor bandage on her arm for the rest of her life. The doctors know now how much we need our lymph nodes and they don't take as many.

When I came around, I asked, "Will I be able to go home tomorrow?" The doctor told me, "Yes - if you get up three times in the night you can go home in the morning." He was joking but I didn't know that – so I made sure I got up three times in the night, and I made sure the nurses recorded it. When the doctor came round to see me in the morning, I reminded him of his promise. He laughed, but he let me go home.

Before I left the hospital that morning, my daughter Tammy brought her daughter – my granddaughter - Karly to see me. She was eight at the time. Karly and I are very close; I was the first person to hold her after she was born. She was due to go on a camping trip that day, and when she came in to see me, she started crying and saying she wouldn't be able to leave me to go camping. I looked at her and said, "Karly, you are going camping. I am getting out of here today and I will be fine. Guess who will be at your Grade 12 graduation? Me!"

Ten years later, Karly asked me to be her date at her grad, and I was.

After the surgery, I felt a sense of optimism. I really felt that I could beat this thing.

And then started the pressure to have chemo and radiation. I had known as soon as I was diagnosed that I would never have either. I don't know how I knew, I just did. It was a kind of sixth sense.

There was a day I remember, sometime after I had been diagnosed, when I was flitting around the house, with the TV on in the background. I rarely had the TV on in the house, but that day, suddenly, there was a show on and the guest was Dr Lorraine Day. She had fought cancer naturally, and was on this show up against doctors and an audience full of cancer sufferers, all of whom had been treated with conventional treatment. It was her against almost every person in the studio. They ripped her apart.

Now I decided I had to get a hold of Dr Day. There were very few people around at that time who supported alternative treatment of cancer, and I felt that she was the one person who would understand. I found the number of her office, and as I dialled, I felt a surge of hope. But there was no answer. I stood in my hallway, and let the phone ring maybe 40 times, wondering what I would do now. Finally a guy picked up and barked down the phone, "Who is this?" I said, "Who is *this*?" He said that he was Dr Day's publicist. He told me they were in the midst of moving offices and that he wasn't even going to take the call. I said, "Well you did, and I need to speak to Dr Day." I told him I had watched the show, and that I wanted to fight my cancer the same way she had.

The publicist said, "Wow. I wasn't happy with her for doing that show. I said she was never again to do a show like that. And she told me, if I help just one person, that's all that matters to me. Out of all the people in the States, we get a call from Canada, and it's you."

He told me he would send me all her DVDs, which he did. I received them three days later. Those DVDs – full of information on alternative treatments - gave me such hope. After watching them, I just knew that I could do it the same way.

Almost immediately after being diagnosed, I started having Vitamin C drips. Before I was even diagnosed, I had been to a lecture in Vancouver by Dr Linus Pauling. He had espoused the benefits of Vitamin C in cancer treatment. The words I remember him saying are, "The first thing I would ever do if I was diagnosed with cancer is to have Vitamin C drips." That stuck with me, and I'm glad it did.

I went to the clinic to have the Vitamin C treatment five days a week right up until when I went to Mexico in the October. I planned my daughter Lori's wedding while I was there. The treatment was expensive. It was like a job; one that I paid for. I would leave home every day at 8am, so I could get there at 9 and try to be first in line, and I would sit there for hours. It was my first glimpse of real death. I saw a lot of people who were using alternative methods as a last resort. It was tough; I watched beautiful young girls sitting beside me, planning their funerals.

I watched them go through the range of emotions that come with cancer: denial, then anger, then acceptance.

I thought, "Holy shit, this is not for me. I am not ready to die."

I knew I wanted to give this fight everything I had. When I got back the report on my blood work, my real body age was 73. I was 52. It was because my body had been fighting cancer for 12 years without me even knowing it. When I looked back, I realised my body was trying to tell me something. I used to get bad colds all the time, sometimes with mucus pouring out of me. I should have paid more attention to my body.

But I was otherwise healthy. Despite being a previous smoker and heavy drinker, I had quit everything over 20 years before. And I mean everything: one day in 1976, I quit alcohol, smoking, coffee, tea, and red meat - all on the same day.

When I gave up drinking, I learned one hugely important lesson: live one day at a time, and if that was too much – live one moment at a time. I think this is true of so many life situations: grief, hardship, addiction, over-eating, illness...

And that is how I handled the cancer. Using that philosophy, I just kept living every day not only at a time but to its fullest. I decided not to keep thinking ahead. I especially chose not to think about the what-ifs.

My youngest daughter Shannon begged me to have chemo. Her friend was going through it at the time and was undergoing every conventional treatment available to her.

I told Shannon, "I'm not doing it. It's my body, and I just cannot put all that poison in me. What I need to do is to make my immune system strong so that I can fight this." Everyone thought I was crazy.

I firmly believe in second opinions. A friend of mine was diagnosed with breast cancer just before she was going away to Hawaii for her 25th wedding anniversary. She came to me, understandably distraught, saying she wasn't going to go to Hawaii. I told her two things: get a second opinion, and go to Hawaii. My feeling was that if it was a tumour, it would still be there when she came back. She went to Hawaii, and when she came back, she got her second opinion – and discovered that the first diagnosis had been wrong. It wasn't breast cancer after all.

I also told my cousin to get a second opinion after she was diagnosed with breast cancer. They wanted to do a mastectomy right away. When she got a second opinion, it wasn't cancer.

I didn't get a second opinion, but then I knew in my heart that I had a tumour.

It was a few weeks after my mastectomy, a rainy Friday afternoon in Vancouver, when I went to my appointed oncologist; a well-renowned doctor who was appalled when I told her that I wanted to treat my cancer naturally. She would not listen. I told her, "This is what I want to do and this is how I want to do it."

She looked at me, obviously confused, and said, "Suzie. For your sisters coming behind you, I want you to try this new chemotherapy." She had already called in a nurse who was busily inserting a needle into my arm; taking a blood test for my compatibility with this "new chemotherapy" that I was not having.

In my head, I was thinking, "Fuck you!" What, in fact, came out of my mouth was: "Actually, what you want is for me to be your guinea pig, so you can see how much chemo you can give me before it kills me." It was not going to be me. I would not allow her to push this new treatment on me.

Incidentally, that "new" form of chemo is not used any more.

She was angry, insulted, incredulous. I guess not many people challenged her. She looked at me as I was leaving and said, "You've got six months to live." It was a terrifying statement, and I stopped, frozen at the door, to digest the words. I took a few deep breaths and walked out. I did not look back.

My shock and fear turned to anger as I was leaving; the prognosis made me even more determined to prove her wrong.

Before I got into the elevator to go home, I announced loudly and dramatically to anyone who would listen that I would never return to that hospital. I may have shouted, "I am NEVER returning to this (insert swear word) hospital, ever!"

Unfortunately, five minutes later, I was back. I had got into the elevator and noticed blood running down my arm, from when they had opened up a vein whilst doing the blood test. I had to go back and sheepishly ask a nurse to attend to it.

By the time I got home that day, I was on fire. I felt that no-one had listened to me; no-one had wanted to hear me. It was their way or no way. In retrospect, I am glad I became so full of anger, because I had a renewed drive and determination to show the oncologists what I could do. I unleashed The Power of Suzie.

After that day, Gary and I made a pact not to tell a soul that I had been handed this 'death sentence'. I didn't want my girls to know or to suffer. In my experience, people look at you differently when they know you have cancer, even more so when they know you have been given a time limit. Friends don't know what to say to you. Some people can't deal with it.

When I did finally tell someone about the six month prognosis, it was long after the six months had passed.

I am strong, but I do my crying on my own. Sometime after being handed that death sentence, I was driving wildly through the streets of Surrey, crying my eyes out, speeding and wondering what would happen to me. Elvis accompanied me, belting out, "How Great Thou Art" at full volume. I didn't cry in front of anyone, even Gary, but I did cry in front of the cop who stopped me that day. As my window went down, I was bawling, with Elvis blaring in the background.

"Did you know you were speeding?" the cop asked me.

"Did you know I've got breast cancer and I've been given six months to live?" I shouted through my tears. The cop really didn't look like he wanted to deal with a hysterical, speeding Elvis freak. "Just go!" he said, and walked away. I'm not sure whether to thank the cop, or Elvis, for getting me off that ticket.

I faced a lot of criticism. My brother came to me one day and screamed at me for 20 minutes; I am not sure what he was saying but I do remember this: "Who do you think you are, not doing chemo?" This was a diabetic man who lived on cola and sugar.

I was weak anyway, and now I had to face my brother's anger. I am sure he had good intentions, but I wasn't having it. We were standing in my kitchen and I calmly said, "Come here," and walked him to the door. He stepped through it, I closed the door and locked it behind him. I didn't have it in me to argue. Our relationship never really recovered after that. He was mad at me because I wouldn't do chemo, and I was mad at him because he didn't take his health seriously. He died in 1999.

My parents were supportive, but my mom did say to me at one point that she thought I should consider doing chemo. She said to me sweetly one day, "You know, I've been talking to my sisters and we really think you should do that chemotherapy thing." My response was "Are you kidding mother?"

I was absolutely determined in my belief, and she accepted it. I think maybe she just felt she had to say it.

I had no idea what would happen to me, I didn't know where this journey would take me. The only thing I knew for certain is that my two year old grandson Triston had saved my life that day. However much of that life I had left, I was determined to fight – for his sake, and for my other grandchildren. I was determined that those kids would know who their crazy grandma was. And they do.

But my fight was only just beginning.

CHAPTER TWO
HEARTBREAK HOTEL

"I am the creator of my experience. I take what I have and make what I want."

—Alan Cohen

I booked a trip to Mexico almost immediately. *Was this really the time for a few weeks lounging around on a beach?* I hear you ask. Well, no, it wasn't. It was time to fight for my life. I am not sure where I got the idea to go to the Gerson Clinic. I already knew that Germany was advanced in cancer treatment, and when I heard, through my research, that the clinic was set up by the daughter of the German physician Max Gerson, I had an instinctive feeling that it was the right thing to do.

There was a slight problem. That problem was money. Three and a half weeks at the Gerson cost $27,000. Gary and I had a successful business but we didn't have $27,000 sitting around. I have to say, this problem didn't bother me too much. I was going anyway. Maybe if one has this kind of resolute determination, money comes. It certainly came to me.

Gary and I had never invested in stocks and bonds; it wasn't our thing. But sometime earlier, a really good friend of ours, Billy, had come to us and suggested we invest $3000 in a seed stock. Gary and I talked about it, and eventually decided that we trusted Billy enough to give it a shot.

On the day of Billy and his wife Marjorie's wedding anniversary – August 23rd – we all went to the States, so the boys could golf and the girls could lunch. That day, I handed Billy a $3000 cheque for the seed stock. Billy was going to pass it on to his broker friend after we returned to Canada. Gary and Billy were on the third hole when Billy swung his club, said, "Uh-oh," and dropped dead. He had had a fatal heart attack. We were, naturally, devastated. Billy's body had to stay in the States that night until we could make arrangements to bring him back to Canada. Our cheque was in his pocket that whole time.

After we got back to Canada, we got the cheque back. Even though we were meant to have the money for the seed stock paid that day – August 23rd - the broker handling the transaction said that, in the circumstances, he would allow us to pay it late. So, in honour of Billy, we made sure we got the cheque to the broker. And then we sat back and waited. We watched, amazed, as it grew and grew, until the day we cashed it in – at $27,000; the exact amount we needed for the Gerson. All I can say is: thanks Billy.

On the day we left for Mexico, my best friend Vicky phoned my girls and said, "Who does your mother think she is, not doing chemo?" It was a few years later that she was diagnosed with colon cancer. I wanted so desperately to help her through it - my way - but she chose to do chemo and radiation. She died six years ago.

I understand people's choices to go the conventional route. I get it. Doctors have been studying cancer for many years. But my frustration comes from a lack of true understanding. People should do their research. They should choose what is right for them, only after they have done that research. I always tell people that the conventional route will always be there – but consider giving the natural route a try first.

I was never going to do chemo or radiation – never. I just knew I could not have bombarded my body with that poison. I wanted to give it every chance I could to be strong. People use holistic therapy as a last resort instead of a first resort. I used it first.

I didn't know how my girls felt about me going to Mexico; I never asked them. Hard headed woman that I was, nothing would have stopped me. Gary knew better than to argue. He came with me to Mexico and supported me throughout the whole experience. If I had had an army of doctors telling me not to do it my way, and if my family had been standing beside them, I still would have chosen this way.

Out of all the conventional doctors I came across in that time, there was only one who seemed to understand me. I don't think he really agreed with my choices, but instead of making me feel small and stupid, he said to me, "Suzie, you're gonna do what you're gonna do. And to be honest, there's a 50-50 chance either way."

So, in early October, we flew into San Diego. We stayed in a beautiful hotel by the ocean, and that night Gary and I went out to a stunningly expensive Mexican restaurant for "my last supper." I knew what was coming over the ensuing months, and I knew it didn't include delicious Mexican meals.

The next morning, a driver came in a van to pick us up from our hotel to take us into Mexico to the sleazy little border town Tijuana. As we crossed the border, I remember Gary looking at me as if to say "What the hell are we doing?" I smiled at him; I still had no doubts that what we were doing was absolutely the right thing.

We pulled into the compound and were met with armed guards at the front of a nondescript but imposing building. If we were in any doubt that this place was a little unconventional, our doubts were soon confirmed.

A female Mexican doctor met us at the door, and seemed overwhelmingly happy to see me. She was babbling away excitedly in Spanish, hugging me, and taking our bags all at once, and I said to her impatiently, "I don't understand! What are you saying?" In perfect English, she said, "For once God has sent me one who hasn't done chemo or radiation. I have a chance with you."

I was so moved by those words. That was the first doctor who had made me feel that there was a chance I would survive. I had been quietly brave, but alone, and lonely, in my resolve - until then.

The nurse hustled us in, our bags were taken from us, and suddenly, it was just us; Gary and I, standing in a clinic in Mexico, not knowing what we would face.

In Canada, I had been told by the doctors that I was stage IV, even though I believed I was Stage III (I always know better than the doctors!)... but at that time, I wrongly believed there was a Stage V. So I think my unwillingness to accept that I was Stage IV was because I wanted to believe it was not as bad as it could have been.

On that first morning in Mexico, they did a live blood analysis and that was the day that I found out there was no Stage V. Stage IV was as bad as it could get. And the Gerson confirmed what the doctors at home had already told me; I was Stage IV. That was quite a lot to take in, all before lunch on our first day.

At lunch time, we were shown to the dining room - poor Gary was not happy when he saw what he would be having for lunch! I can't remember exactly what we had that day, but of course it would have been pure, healthy, clean food. Although we had always eaten what we believed was a healthy diet, we had no idea what that really meant until we went to the Gerson.

We found a table and sat down with the other patients who had been waiting for us to arrive – we were the last arrivals of the day.

There were three couples sitting at the table. One of the women said "Hello," and then, "Don't tell us anything yet! We have been playing a game... as people walk in, we have been guessing who has the cancer and who is the companion." Most of the time, the group was split 50/50 on their guesses. With us, one hundred per cent of them guessed that Gary was the patient. I guess I did look healthy. I was not a skinny woman. I had all my hair. My skin was good. I was a picture of robust health. Ironic.

Of course, when I look back now, I realise that Gary was looking sick because he was; he was sick with worry - which explains their analysis.

It's weird to make friends with people who have cancer. There is no preamble; no time wasting; there is a very real sense of time passing, which renders small talk pointless. Friendships get formed very quickly.

After lunch, it was down to business; the business of saving my life. And so began three weeks of intense, pure, dogged hard work.

I was the only one at the clinic who could do the full therapy, because I had never done chemo or radiation. Patients who had undergone conventional treatments could only do four or five juices a day. I was having 13. I was their star patient.

Max Gerson, a German physician, born in Poland in 1881, developed his therapy as a treatment for migraine and TB. In 1928, he began to use it as a treatment for cancer. In 1936 he moved to the States and continued his work as a revolutionary in natural cancer treatment.

When he died in 1959, his daughter Charlotte vowed to continue his work, and in 1977 she founded the Gerson Instutute.

The therapy is based on the treatment of harmful toxins in the body, and involves patients consuming a purely vegetarian diet, drinking up to 13 pure, organic juices per day, dietary supplements, coffee enemas and daily doses of castor oil.

Charlotte Gerson is a passionate and imposing woman. When I met her she was 75 years old, and her eyes were an incredible piercing, clear crystal blue. She has eaten a healthy diet her entire life. Every time I saw her she was eating an apple.

Whilst at the clinic, I befriended two young guys. Gary would go off with their wives to sneak into town to get coffee, something other than Gerson food. I, of course, was getting my coffee fix another way – up my bottom! ("The upside down coffee" as my daughter Shannon describes it now.)

Gary would put on aftershave to go out with these two women. One day I heard a tromp, tromp, tromp, coming down the hallway. One of the nurses said, "Uh-oh, she's mad." Charlotte Gerson marched into my room, and sure enough she was steaming. Aftershave in the Gerson Clinic was strictly forbidden. I had to say, "It wasn't me Charlotte, it was my husband." I wanted to add, "I don't even wear aftershave," but it was clearly not the time for jokes.

Charlotte sat on my bed and told me how important it was not to put chemicals on our bodies, and not to be around chemicals on other bodies either. "We are all cleansing here," she scolded before she left.

As well as the juices, I had a scalding hot bath every other day for around 30 minutes. They bring your body up to a fevered temperature, so that your body fights the fever and kills the cancer cells.

It was a time consuming process. 13 juices a day, five coffee enemas, castor oil, the baths. There were lectures every day. It was intense. The point was to learn to change the terrain of the body, so the cancer doesn't come back. Cancer cannot thrive if the terrain is different.

While I was there, I made friends with a beautiful woman called Cathy who was 42 years old – my daughter Shannon's age now. She had three young kids. She said, "I would never ever have done chemo if I had known what I know now." Being at the Gerson was her last ditch effort to survive. She died two weeks after she left.

I would sit with my new friends and they would say to me, "How did you know not to do chemo?"

I just did.

I was so focused on staying alive that I was like a horse with blinders. I would not claim it – I never gave it a name and I never gave it power. People say "my cancer..." - that's claiming it. For me it was the same as having a cold and doing everything you can to get rid of it.

For the time I was in the clinic, I kept a photo of all of my grandchildren beside me always – to give me a reason to carry on. They were my reason to survive. I believe even now that had a huge role in getting me through.

Two days after I got to the clinic, I called home for my messages. There was a message from my oncologist demanding to know why I hadn't turned up for my chemo session. I thought that was strange, as I had told her firmly I had no intention of doing chemo. But it confirmed what I already knew - she had not listened to a single word.

When I left that clinic three and a half weeks later, I felt fantastically healthy and more importantly, positive; in fact certain that I would be OK. My blood work showed a huge improvement. I left with so much more hope than I had gone with.

When I was coming back through the border from Mexico, I had 20 enema buckets in my luggage. I thought the whole world was going to start doing enemas; I had read so much good information about them. I had boxes and boxes of stuff, including a $3500 juicer. I knew I was way over-loaded. I went to the customs officer and said, "Here's my story. I was just diagnosed with breast cancer. I have been down in Mexico at the Gerson, and this is why I have so much stuff."

He looked at me and said, "Well, you know, when I was a young boy, I was diagnosed with cancer, and I am still here. Go through."

I got home in early November, but I was weak from doing all the juices and enemas. I did the programme for another four months after I got back. It became my way of life. I also became a messenger; a loud and pushy advocate of healthy living. I gave advice, even when unasked for.

I was shopping one day, and saw five guys standing outside Future Shop; they were all smoking. I guess they worked there and it was their break. I walked up to them and said, "Would you guys mind if I shared a story with you?" They looked at me weirdly, as if to say, "Yes we do mind; now go away." But they didn't say a word. I told them I had just returned from Mexico and that I was fighting for my life with cancer, and I told them about my two friends from Mexico; both wealthy, successful businessmen with everything to live for. Both heavy drinkers, both heavy smokers. Both now dead. I felt compelled to share that story with them.

A few weeks later, I was walking into our vacuum store in Langley, and a guy came towards me saying, "Hey! You're that lady from Future Shop. You came over and told us all we should quit smoking!" I was taken aback. Was he mad at me?

He then went on to tell me that he hadn't yet stopped smoking, but he hadn't stopped thinking about what I had said that day. "I am going to quit," he told me. I guess at the risk of upsetting five people, I may have had an impact on one.

I feel like I should be a missionary, sharing my story. That's why I am doing this now.

I carried on doing the juices, castor oil and enemas and living as close to the Gerson lifestyle as I could. My liver was in bad shape, so another thing I would do is make clay packs and put them against my liver, trying to draw out the toxins. I did all of this for four months. I am a people person, and this lifestyle makes it difficult to see people – there's no time for anything else. I stayed in the house a lot. When you're fighting for your life, you do whatever it takes. But it was an all-consuming existence, and it was tough. I hid it - even my girls had no idea what I was going through... although one of my girls was to, sadly, find out later for herself.

I was so determined to get my life back. So much so that I may have run before I could walk. One day I decided to walk into town, but I hadn't realised how weak I was, and halfway there, I became hysterical and broke down. My advice to anyone going through it would be to take it slowly, take it easy; take the time to heal and recover.

I desperately wanted life to be normal again. So that December, we went to Maui. This time we planned to have a holiday. But I still kept doing my enemas. I took wheatgrass. I juiced.

I remember being on the beach, with one flattened breast, and people would stare openly at me. I guess it did look a little weird, but I wouldn't give in to pressure and would not put on my prosthetic. I think I was making a statement, and I think that statement was: "Fuck you cancer!"

Whilst in Maui, I was walking on the beach one day and I saw a lady who I knew from my many trips there. She said, "Suzie, how are you? Have you had a good year?" And I dissolved into tears. I was so happy to see her. I was happy to be there. I was happy to be alive.

That Christmas, my girls bought me a puppy as a surprise; a beautiful golden retriever. I adore dogs, and it was a gorgeous little puppy, but the thought of looking after something other than myself and Gary terrified me. I knew I couldn't keep it. It slept beside me that night, but the next day I had to tearfully tell the girls, "I just can't look after it." It was as much as I could do to look after myself and Gary. But the girls really had no idea what I was going through. I never set out to keep it a secret, I just didn't really broadcast it.

I believe in rituals. I believe in positive thinking. I read everything I could, and I recited prayers and affirmations every day.

One of the rituals I had was to walk on my treadmill every day; as I did so, I would hold my hands above my head and channel the light through my head and into my body, praying to God for the cancer to be gone, and really believing deep in my soul that it was leaving. I would do this religiously every single morning.

And then one day, sometime after Christmas, I was at home alone. It was early evening, and I suddenly realised that I hadn't done my daily ritual on the treadmill. At that moment, I stopped and said to myself, "It's gone."

And I firmly, absolutely, resolutely, believed it had.The ugly, all-consuming, terrible, terrifying thing they call cancer - had gone.

CHAPTER THREE
Have I told you lately that I love you?

"Keep your faith in beautiful things; in the sun when it is hidden, in the spring when it is gone."

—Roy R Gibson

Mine was a comfortable upbringing, typical of that generation – with hard working, loving parents, two brothers, a sister and a nomadic lifestyle that took us all over Canada as we were growing up.

I was a wartime baby, born in Winnepeg, Manitoba on May 26th 1945 to a Canadian mother and a second-generation Irish father (my dad's dad was Irish). I had two older brothers, Michael and Richard, and seven years after I was born, along came my baby sister Sharon.

My dad was in sales and we moved around a lot growing up; this gave me a gypsy spirit which I still have – much to husband Gary's disgust (he is a home body).

Every summer as a child we would head to our family cottage by the lake, and stay there for the entire summer. It was idyllic. There were always lots of people around, with cousins coming and going. To this day, I can still recall the sound of the water lapping against the shore as I fell asleep. Those summers, I believe, helped create a strong family bond that balanced the moving around, and provided me with some cherished family memories.

My mother always kept beautiful gardens – she had a love for flowers which I inherited – and in summer, even now, I am happiest when surrounded by colourful blooms.

My mom was a meat, potatoes and vegetables kind of cook, with big Sunday dinners with homemade desserts. Her homemade chocolate cake was legendary. It was a comfort food for me, even after I left home. There was no junk food around when we were growing up, and a Coke in our house was rare. I am grateful for that.

I remember when the first pancake house opened up where we were living at the time. Dad came home late that night and announced that we were all going out for pancakes. It was unheard of and we were all so excited.

My parents were loving and I had a happy childhood, but it wasn't perfect. My dad was a drinker, a hazard of his experience in the war. He had never touched alcohol before going off to war. But when he came back, so Mom told us, he was a changed man.

When he was in England during war time, one day, he and his good friend from Winnepeg were out on an army exercise; they were on motorcycles following an army truck. They would always ride in the same formation, one on each side at the rear of the trucks. On this day, for the first time ever, and for no apparent reason, my dad and his friend switched sides; Dad on the right and his mate on the left.

But on this day there was a terrible accident. The truck stopped suddenly, without warning, and my dad's friend crashed his motorcycle into the back of the truck. My dad watched as his friend was decapitated. My dad started drinking after that.

After his return, Dad became a car salesman, and he and Mom started various businesses. Later, my parents bought a beautiful horse breeding farm in Aldergrove, BC. It was called Shadowland.

In the summer of 1971, I was visiting Mom at the farm. She was sitting up on a fence, and we were watching the horses run in the fields. She said calmly to me, "Suzie, feel this lump." I did - it was the size of a pea - and so it all began, for her, myself and later my daughter Shannon – breast cancer came into our lives.

My Mom had very large breasts (40E) and her whole life would wish them to be smaller.

Be careful what you wish for.

In those days, breast cancer was treated aggressively, and my Mom had a radical treatment, starting with a single mastectomy. Because she was so large, they couldn't even out the flat side, and the weight on one side was making her walk crookedly and was affecting her back. So they removed the other breast too.

My Mom handled her diagnosis and operation with dignity and grace, the way she did everything in her life. I can't say the same for my father and me. On the day of her operation, we were both emotional wrecks. This was in my drinking days, and the two of us were a mess. We got a call from the hospital to tell us surgery was over, so we hopped into my little convertible and headed to the hospital. We must have looked a sight as we arrived there, drunk, with our wild hair and crying hysterically. My poor mother – who never took a drop of alcohol her entire life – had to endure her husband and daughter, these crazy Irish drinkers, out of control by her hospital bed. The nurses eventually asked us to leave.

She never worried about getting her breasts rebuilt, and she never had any other treatment, as far as I know. She did that right.

My mother was an entrepreneur and a visionary. She wrote a book "Family Story" which she typed, bound and distributed to our family, and in it, the story of her life shows what a strong, re-sourceful woman she was. Her and my father had several success-ful businesses, whilst bringing up four children, breeding race horses, building, buying and selling properties, and going through illness.

In her book, she writes:

"In the fall (of '86), Susan and I went to San Diego to the Health Institute. We had read the founder Ann Wigmore's book "*Why Suffer*" many years before, and were eager to be enlightened. It was while we were in San Diego that we learned of a cancer sufferer who had cured her colon cancer by the use of wheatgrass. We were so impressed with the benefits of wheatgrass."

Little was known about wheatgrass at the time, but Ann Wigmore knew about it, and so did my Mom.

When I met Gary at age 20, I fell for his charm, good looks and humour. We met in a bar in Vancouver. His friend had tried to chat me up, but it was Gary who succeeded in getting my number. Our courtship was brief and marriage was an easy decision for two people who were deeply in love. We went on to build a good solid life for ourselves, with four beautiful daughters, Lori, Tammy, Daaynna and Shannon. But somewhere along the way, we lost ourselves to alcohol. I can't say how it happened; it was a slow progression, but before I knew it, Gary and I were both drinking regularly. We loved to party.

I had started drinking at an early age, but I don't think I had a problem with it until I was a young mother. I could go all week without it, but by Thursday or Friday, I was ready to go, hard. I would start drinking at home before I went out, and would say to myself "I will only have three drinks," but the third would inevitably lead to a fourth, fifth and more, and I would lose control.

One night at my parent's house, my sister and I sat up all night drinking. My parents owned a racehorse that had won a big race down in California, and we thought it would be a good idea to bring him into the living room. Onto the shag carpet. My poor Mom! That was my first major blackout. I couldn't tell you one thing that I remember about that night. It scared the living daylights out of me.

Another thing that scared me was how out of shape I was. I re-member being in a curling bonspiel with these three older women - neighbours - none of whom drank or smoked. There was me, 20 years younger, brought in as a spare - a smoker and a drinker - and we kept winning our games, even though we were supposed to be a losing team. So I had to keep playing. I kept thinking, "When will this end?" I just didn't have the stamina that they did.

There was another night I can remember, when I started to sus-pect that things had to change. Gary and I were at a party in the States, and my good friend "Softly" was visiting from England. Af-ter a few drinks, I started to think that some guy was being rude to Softly, and out of the blue, I punched this guy and laid him out; there was blood everywhere. The guy stood up, wobbly on his feet, and suddenly my brother, who was also at the party, appeared. He accused this guy of attacking his sister, and promptly laid another punch on this poor, innocent man. It was mayhem.

I said to Gary, "We gotta get out of here." We piled into the car, with me driving. I was so drunk that I could hardly see straight. I was doing 100 miles an hour up the freeway back to Canada.

We hit a patch of ice and I almost lost control of the car; it was so bad that Gary awoke from his drunken stupor and said, "What the hell is going on?" I don't know how we didn't die that night.

In the cold light of the next day, we both agreed how crazy we had been, and it scared us. But still we kept drinking.

And then, there was one awful day that changed everything. One Christmas Eve, I had a drinking session that lasted most of the night. I was around 30, and married with three girls living at home. I woke in the morning to a pounding head and a stern looking Gary standing over me. He said, "The girls are waiting outside for Santa." I had hidden the gifts the night before, in a drunken daze, and couldn't remember where.

In my now hungover haze, I stood up and looked out of the win-dow, and there they were, the three girls, waiting by the side of the road for Santa to arrive. It broke my heart and it still does. I couldn't tell this story for years.

Gary had me walking around the fields, snow crunching underfoot, drinking coffee and trying to sober me up. The horses were following me and nudging my arm as if to say, "Come on, sober up!"

We finally found the presents on top of a shed.

I knew then that I had a problem. I carried on drinking until February of the following year, but I never got drunk again. I didn't quit right away, because alcoholics need time to accept their problem.

But then, on Valentine's Day in 1976, I quit. I was 31 years old. I have an addictive personality and I knew it was all or nothing. I gave up smoking, coffee, tea, red meat, and alcohol... all in one day. Overnight. I have never gone back to any of it since that day.

Gary continued the drinking lifestyle, but his days were numbered. Recovering alcoholics cannot live with active alcoholics. I told Gary that I would leave him if he continued drinking, and I meant it.

One day in March, I got a call from some girls at a party to say my husband was there. He had just smoked three jumbo joints, was drunk as could be, and was just getting in the car to drive home. He somehow made it, but he came home to a steaming wife. I picked up a heavy candle holder, the first thing I could lay my hands on. I hit him as hard as I could, left him there and stormed off to bed. The next day I was planning on leaving. But it never came to that, because that was the day Gary quit drinking. He has never touched another drop.

After ten years of a marriage based on alcohol abuse, suddenly we were free. It changed our lives, it changed our marriage. It changed our girls' lives.

I was very close to my parents and losing them devastated me. My dad died while I was away in Florida on a golfing holiday. The day before it happened, it had been a beautiful sunny day. Gary and I were in Alligator Alley and decided to stop at a roadside diner for lunch. As we walked in, my dad's favourite song was playing. It stopped me in my tracks for some reason.

That night I had a bad dream. It woke me up, and I remember being in the bathroom and saying to Gary, "My dad's gone." I just knew it. Gary suggested that I call home but I didn't. I was fending off the pain I knew was coming my way.

The next morning, we came back from breakfast to find a light flashing on the answerphone in the hotel room. I said to Gary, "Please don't check that." And I went down to the pool.

Gary came down shortly after that, and I knew from his face that he had checked the answerphone message. My dad had died.

That was the only time I have been tempted to drink again. There was a bar right there by the pool, and as I sat crying my eyes out, I felt that the only way I could numb the pain was with alcohol. I resisted.

When we got to the airport the next day, Gary collapsed at the airport. We didn't know it, but he had severe IBS. He was in excruciating pain, curled up on the airport floor in the foetal position. They didn't want us to fly but I insisted. On the plane home, I wrote a fabulous eulogy to my dad, which I ended up reading out at the funeral (despite being terrified of public speaking).

Within that 11 months, my dad died, Gary got sick, was in hospital for 4 months, my friend Vicky died, and my friend Bonny died. Bonny was my sponsor in AA, she was my mentor and like a second mother to me. After she died, I remember saying to my mother, "The worst thing that could happen now, Mom, is that something happens to you." We laughed about that, and then a month later she died. She was 86, and it was a terrible time for my family and me, but I can't deny that she'd had a full and happy life.

I lost two angels that year, one in March and the other in April. But I feel blessed to have had them in my life.

We had a service for Mom, which happened to fall on Mother's Day, and afterwards, her grand-children and great-children scattered her ashes in the stream than ran through her beloved Shadowland, where we all had so many happy family memories. She would have been so pleased.

There is a prayer which I carry with me to this day. It's from Al-Anon, where I went when I had given up alcohol and Gary was still drinking. I feel it applies to what I am trying to say in this book.

Just For Today

Just for today I will try to live through this day only, and not tackle all my problems at once. I can do something for twelve hours that would appall me if I felt that I had to keep it up for a lifetime.

Just for today I will be happy. This assumes to be true what Abraham Lincoln said, that "Most folks are as happy as they make up their minds to be."

Just for today I will adjust myself to what is, and not try to adjust everything to my own desires. I will take my 'luck' as it comes, and fit myself to it.

Just for today I will try to strengthen my mind. I will study. I will learn something useful. I will not be a mental loafer. I will read something that requires effort, thought and concentration.

Just for today I will exercise my soul in three ways: I will do somebody a good turn, and not get found out; if anybody knows of it, it will not count. I will do at least two things I don't want to do – just for exercise. I will not show anyone that my feelings are hurt; they may be hurt, but today I will not show it.

Just for today I will be agreeable. I will look as well as I can, dress becomingly, keep my voice low, be courteous, criticize not one bit. I won't find fault with anything, nor try to improve or regulate anybody but myself.

Just for today I will have a program. I may not follow it exactly... but I will have it. I will save myself from two pests: hurry and indecision.

Just for today I will have a quiet half hour all by myself, and relax. During this half hour, sometime, I will try to get a better perspective of my life.

Just for today I will be unafraid. Especially I will not be afraid to enjoy what is beautiful, and to believe that as I give to the world, so the world will give to me.

CHAPTER FOUR
Make the World Go away

"Doubt whom you will, but never yourself."

—*Christine Bovee*

In 1999, I found another lump. This time the lump was on my left breast. This new discovery was...inconvenient, because I knew I would have to get it tested. Really? I have to go through this again? The doctor's appointments... the biopsy...the waiting...the creeping doubt...

Except, this time, I had no doubts. I wasn't worried about it, I knew I was doing the right things for my body and I didn't for one second think this new lump could be cancerous.

At the first doctor's appointment, before it was even diagnosed, my doctor said to me, "You are going to have to have the breast off." Was there a glimpse of self-righteousness in her eyes?

I ignored her. I was getting good at ignoring doctors.

They tested it, and five weeks later I got a call from my pessimist doctor to say that the lump wasn't cancerous. Was there a touch of annoyance in her voice? I calmly, and maybe a little smugly, said, "No...I didn't think it was."

I know I seem casual, but it's because I really never doubted myself. I think we know our own bodies better than doctors do. But it is a little scary to me that there could be people out there having surgery and treatment, at the behest of their doctors, when they don't really need it. Be aware of your body; be aware of your choices, that's all I am saying.

That little hiccup out the way, it was time to think about reconstruction of my right breast. The specialist I was referred to suggested I have a tram flap operation. It sounded so easy, so simple, and I took her word for it that it was the right thing to do. It wasn't. I didn't even really think about it or research it; I was trusting. I know, that doesn't sound like me, does it? This doctor said to me, "Suzie, you are a perfect candidate for this operation. It can be very painful, but I know you have a high pain tolerance."

That should have been my first clue to just up and run.

In that tauntingly arrogant thing called retrospect, this is one doctor I should have also ignored. But I was vain, like most women. I wanted breasts. I wanted a *pair* of breasts; I certainly didn't want a single.

This operation involves taking the stomach muscles, hoisting them up and making a breast from that muscle fibre. Piece of cake, right? Wrong. Not a piece of cake; a piece of my body that was being put somewhere it didn't want to be. But of course, I didn't know that yet.

I was determined to do it; it seemed like a really good and obvious solution. On the day of the operation, I remember being cheery and quite hopeful; I was going to war again; this time to get back to looking like a woman.

As I was being prepped for the operation, Gary said to me, "Please, I beg you with all my heart, get your clothes on and let's go home." He had a gut feeling, and I should have listened.

I admit, it was vanity that kept me focused on this operation. I had one good breast and one flat one. It just didn't feel right. It certainly didn't look right. I had been struggling with the concept of having a prosthesis for one of them. I just didn't like it. The prosthesis was like a warm jelly, and on a hot day I would feel like it was melting and I would often just pull it right out.

When I regained consciousness from the op, I wanted to die. There was an intolerable burning and searing pain engulfing my body. From the minute I woke up, those muscles were screaming to go back to where they had come from. It was horrific, far worse than I ever imagined.

After that, they kept me in for five days. The recovery was slow and painful. I wouldn't let the girls come and see me. I hate being in hospital – I may have mentioned that already – and when Gary arrived to visit me on the sixth day, I had my bags packed and I was sitting on the edge of the bed. I told him I was going home. I hadn't been discharged, but I was adamant. Gary was concerned; he hesitated, looking around the room for a nurse or doctor. I said, "I don't care if you take me or not. If you won't take me, I'll get a cab."

That night was a nightmare. I realised that I hadn't had a bowel movement since the operation, and they had given me nothing to prompt one. When I got home, I made myself a fresh natural juice, and sometime after that, I found myself in the bathroom, screaming. I was having that bowel movement alright – and it was stuck. Sorry for the explicitness, but that's what happened, and it led to something even worse.

As I was screaming, and pushing, and crying, I felt a pop, pop, pop – it was my stitches popping open. Everything seemed to come undone.

To be honest, I was more concerned about the bowel movement issue than the popping. That on its own was pretty excruciating – but Gary came to my rescue. I won't go into too much detail here, but he pulled that thing out of me. Now that, my friends, is true love.

It was three weeks before the hospital could get me in to repair the damage that the bowel movement caused. In the meantime, I

had a big hernia sticking out of my stomach. It was a really difficult time, living with, and accepting, the after-effects of an operation that I had opted for in the name of vanity. It just wasn't worth
it.

In May of that year, we took a trip to New York. It was too soon
to travel, but you gotta live your life – as you know by now, I
firmly believe that. We were at the Empire State Building, walking
down the stairs, when I felt another popping sound. It came undone again. What were they using for these stitches? Cotton
thread? Whatever it was, it wasn't strong enough to hold me together. Did I need some kind of super-strength fishing line? Rope?
Heavy duty cables?

When I got back home to Canada, I got re-stitched again and
was referred back to the surgeon. She said to me, "I am so sorry
about this. I don't know what to do." That didn't really inspire
much confidence. She referred me to another doctor, whom I could
only hope did know what to do.

He examined me and told me that they would have to put surgi-
cal mesh into my body to hold everything together. It didn't seem
far off the fishing line/rope concept.

As I was leaving the new doctor's office, he called me back and
said, "Suzie. You need to know there are no guarantees. I will try
my best, but I don't know if it will work." That didn't inspire much
confidence either, but by now, I had no choice. The hernia was still
sticking right out of my stomach, and I knew something had to be
done.

So I had the mesh installed, and it's in my body to this day. For
two weeks after the op, I could not even lift a purse, or a carton of
milk. I would go up, and come down stairs, on my rear end.

The result today is that I am a mess down there. My colon has
prolapsed as the muscle that was holding it in place is not there
anymore. My bladder is not functioning properly, and the scar tissue is excessive. The lady who gets to work on trying to rectify

this problem now (she manipulates my stomach with her hands to break down the scar tissue) says she has never seen anyone as bad.

I was only supposed to wear a compression girdle for a few weeks after the op, but 12 years later, I still cannot live without one.

I can sometimes be sitting – reading a book or eating dinner - and I feel a tugging sensation, like that muscle is still fighting to go back to where it should be. After all these years.

I just want everything back to where it was supposed to be. Seven years ago, I asked a different doctor if the op could be reversed. I think I may have begged him a little. He looked at me with fear in his eyes and said, "You're a can of worms and I don't want to touch you." He might as well have gone running from the room, with his hands over his head, screaming, "Don't make me go in there!"

I figured then that I would have to live with it, and I have had no other option – but in the past few years, it's got worse. It is sometimes intolerable.

It's the worst decision I have ever made. I implore anyone who is facing breast reconstruction surgery – do not do what I did. Or at least think seriously about it. If you are considering reconstruction surgery, my advice to you is to please consider your options carefully. If possible, look into stem cell surgery.

If I knew then what I know now, I wouldn't have had any surgery, not even the mastectomy. I know, with the right guidance, that the body is capable of eating tumours. Surgery is drastic and can lead to more complications. I even believe that it can lead to the cancer spreading in the body. So, again, with that lovely, self-satisfied little thing called retrospect, if I had to do it all again I know that my decisions would be different. And today, I am certain that I wouldn't be held together with something that could probably net a 50 pound shark.

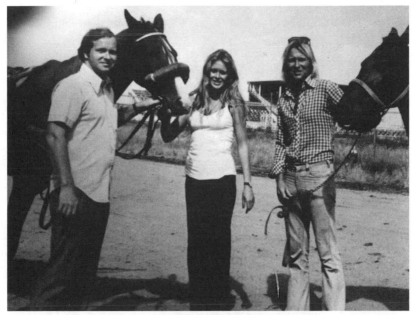

My brothers and sister: Richard, Sharon and Michael

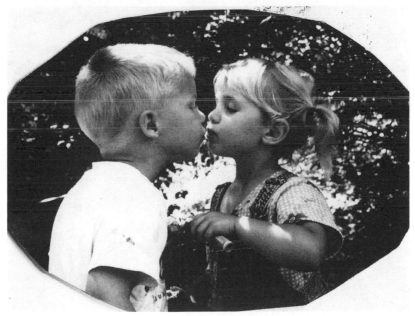

Grandchildren Triston and Brooklyn – when they were both two years old

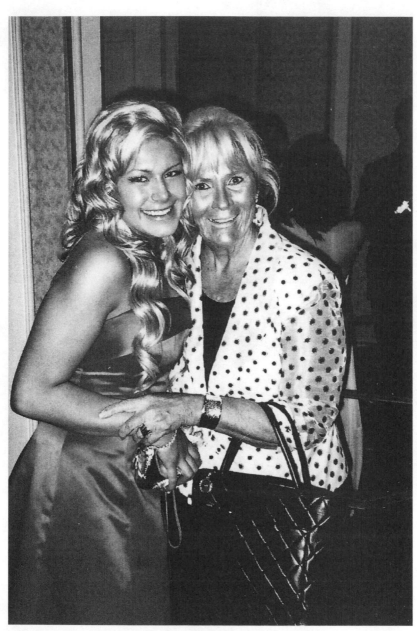

Grand-daughter Karly and I, taken at her
Grade 12 Grad at the Vancouver Hotel

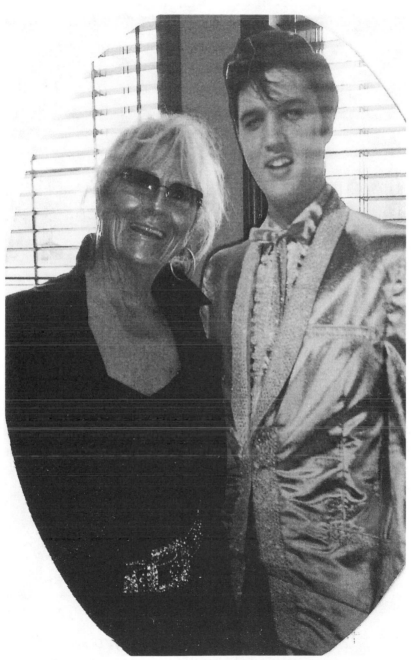

Elvis and I – unfortunately this was just a cardboard cut-out!

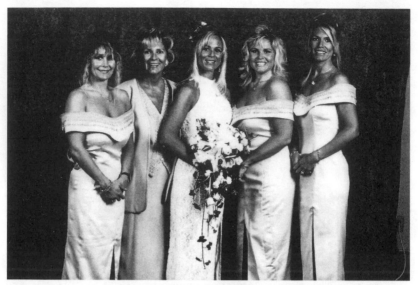

Steve and Shannon`s wedding reception.
The girls and I
Left to right: Lori, me, Shannon, Daaynna and Tammy

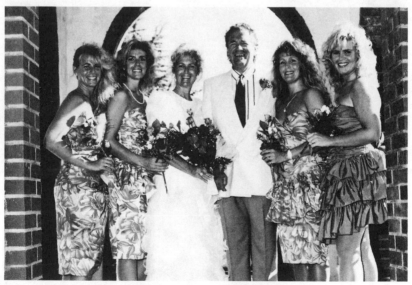

Our 25th wedding anniversary
Left to right: Shannon, Tammy, me, Gary, Lori, Daaynna
One of the happiest days of my life

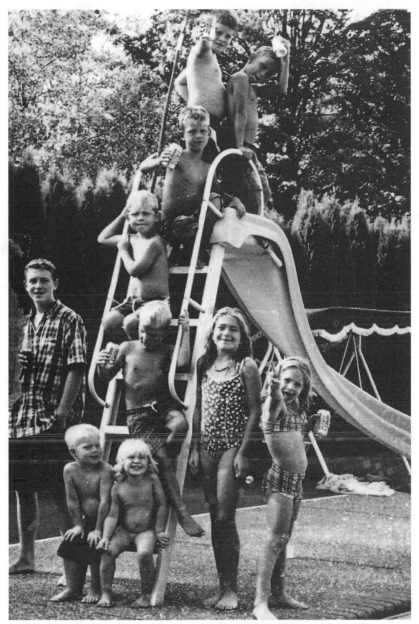

The Grandchildren by the pool – taken on the day Triston found the lump
Left to right: Nephew Danny, Grandkids Triston, Brooklyn, Beau, Tanner,
Mitchell, Talyor, Kodie, Karly, Krisdee

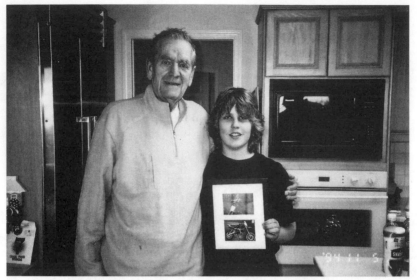

Gary with Grandson Tanner at Tanner's 13th Birthday party in 2005.
Gary was very sick at the time.

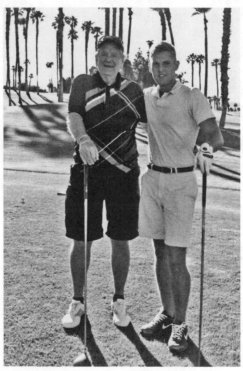

Gary with Grandson Tanner, golfing in Palm Desert in 2012

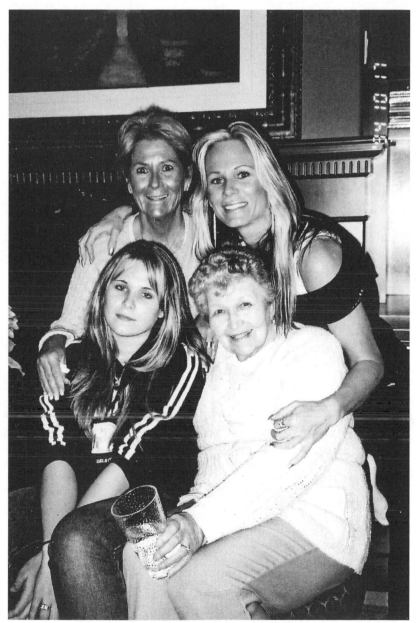

With Grandma Val:
Left to right: Me, Shannon, Krisdee, Mom

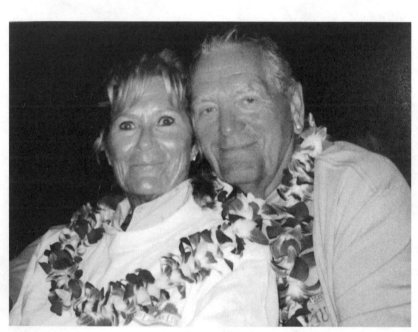

Gary and I

CHAPTER FIVE

HELP ME MAKE IT THROUGH THE NIGHT

"My happiness depends on me, I choose joy now."

—Alan Cohen

In 2003, Gary was diagnosed with prostate cancer. He had never had any symptoms; it just showed up in his blood work. We were never really concerned about it and he never once considered having any conventional treatment. We knew we could beat it on our own.

Then in 2005, he was suffering from nausea and extreme back ache and he developed a severe case of IBS. He was taken into hospital to have his colon removed. Whilst on the operating table, his colon burst and he almost died. He spent the next five months in hospital. He was very sick and very weak.

Whilst he was in hospital, it was my 60th birthday. I decided to take the girls and a few friends to a local winery (even though I don't drink, I still love wineries). I was wearing a cute white skirt suit.

We had a lovely day, but I didn't feel quite right, and by the time I got home, my white skirt was covered in blood. Prior to this time, I had been getting some spotting but not enough to worry about. It was no big deal, or so I thought. To be honest, I thought it was a hormonal issue. I ignored the white suit incident, though sadly that lovely suit never saw the light of day again. It was ruined.

I should have been listening to my body, but I was consumed with everything else that was going on at the time and with Gary being sick.

One night a few weeks after that, Gary asked me to bring him some mushroom soup. I dutifully arrived at the hospital with the soup, and as he got out of bed to prepare to eat it, I lay in his bed. I was feeling nauseous and tired and was suffering from unusually hot flushes. Yes, definitely hormonal, I thought.

Again, I ignored it, but by the time I got home that night, the car seat was covered in blood. I stumbled into the house, feeling weak and ill, and managed to get myself to bed. All the while, I was pouring with blood, and I noticed clots as well. Then I passed out.

When I awoke, my daughters Daaynna and Shannon and grand-daughters were standing over me. They had been visiting Gary at the hospital and the nurse there told them that she had seen me and thought I was haemorrhaging. They raced right over. Thank God they did, because I really believe I wouldn't have made it otherwise.

It was a bloodbath, with the bed sheets, floor and towels absolutely drenched.

Shannon said, "Mother, you're going to the hospital."

I said, "No, I am staying here in bed."

I am a stubborn woman, have I mentioned that already? But the girls weren't having any of it. Before I knew it, there were three hunky firemen in my house. The girls had called an ambulance, and of course, the fire service came too.

It was a comical trip to the hospital. I was in the back of the ambulance listening to my daughter Daaynna chatting up the driver in the front. Meanwhile, the paramedic in the back with me was panicking. It was the same old story; he couldn't get a vein. I was so weak, and he was struggling to look calm.

When we got to the hospital, they called in the guy who is the Vein Master – I don't know how he did it but he got one.

Whilst waiting to see a doctor, I passed a clot so big that I felt like I was giving birth. A bed pan wouldn't even hold it. They had to get a bucket.

At 1am, after they had stabilised me, and the girls had gone home, they put me in my room. Strangely, it was right next door to Gary's room. The nurse thought I had gone loopy because as she wheeled me passed Gary's room, I said weakly, "Oh – that's my husband's room!"

"No it isn't dear," she said, smiling sweetly.

The next morning, I got out of bed, and in my hospital gown and pulling my IV behind me, I walked into the room next door.

I am a practical joker, and have always played terrible jokes on Gary throughout our marriage. As I stood at the foot of Gary's bed, in the role of the quintessential hospital patient, this time my husband thought I had gone over the top. "Come on, Suzie, why are you doing this?"

"Actually, Gar," I said, "I am here for real. I was admitted last night, and I am in the next room!"

We laughed about that. What else could we do?

A few days later, the biopsy came back and confirmed what I had started to suspect: I had uterine cancer. They later said it wasn't associated with the breast cancer.

Weirdly, I wasn't scared. Once again, I knew what to do. I got it; I had to get rid of it.

They wanted to send me home, but this time I refused. I said, "I have got to get well so I can look after Gary when he comes out." What a pair. "You need to sort this out," I told them, though I wasn't really sure how they could.

They did a full hysterectomy. Two days later, I left to go home; still weak, and perturbed by the diagnosis, but I was determined to get well for Gary. Again, the pressure was on to do chemo and radiation.

As I left the hospital, they said to me, "We will see you when you come back for the chemo and radiation." I said, "Yeah, yeah, yeah," and left. I have never been back. They have never seen me again in that hospital to this day.

Suzie had left the building!

Actually, that's not completely true. They did see me again in that hospital, but only because I was accompanying Gary recently to a doctor's appointment, where he was having a prostate exam. When we walked into the doctor's office (this was the same doctor who had first diagnosed my breast cancer back in '97), he looked up and said to me jokingly, "You are a very bad girl... you were meant to come back here, and I haven't seen you in seven years." He asked what I had done to treat the uterine cancer and I replied, "Nothing. I got my body alkaline." He tut-tutted, so I responded by saying, "I look like I'm dying don't I?"

Five years earlier, just before this doctor took a semi-retirement, he had given a speech in his office about how I was one of his star patients. He had said, "I have five patients that I call my heroes, and you are one of them."

That doctor was always supportive of my choices, but I also think he was a little sceptical of them too.

I knew what I had to do to get Gary and I well again. We had allowed our bodies to become acidic. We both went through a period of drinking copious amounts of fizzy water. We were under the misguided impression that this water was good for us. Wrong! This "water" is not healthy, and is in fact extremely acidic. We had allowed our bodies to become acidic, and we needed to change that.

Any piece of gold jewellery I wore in those days was turning green, so I knew I was going acidic again. It was a sign.

So now we had to change our lifestyles once again. We started to eat an alkaline diet, and we juiced regularly. But it wasn't enough, especially for Gary.

CHAPTER SIX
Only Believe

"Water ionisation could be one of the most important health breakthroughs in our era."

—*Robert G Wright*

Gary was not doing well. His recovery was slow and complicated and it was hard to stay positive in those dark days.

He became withdrawn and sullen and I struggled to cope with his moods. Our whole lives changed.

We decided to sell our vacuum business, a difficult decision but necessary for our health, it seemed.

After doing some research into different treatment options for Gary, we opted to go to Newport Beach to a treatment centre run by the well-known Dr Whittaker. We went essentially to deal with Gary's heart arrhythmia, which was worrying me greatly.

Gary undertook a series of treatments involving hyperbaric chambers, chelation, and Vitamin C drips, as well as lectures and education.

I would go to the lectures with Gary; I wanted to learn as much as I could. At one of the meetings after dinner, Dr Whittaker announced to the class that there was a lady in the room who had beaten cancer without using drugs. I didn't even realise he was talking about me. He said to the room, "Stand up and applaud her." He then looked at me and told me he was proud of me for beating cancer naturally. Dr Whittaker! I felt pretty proud of myself that day.

We spent three weeks at the treatment centre. It was an expensive endeavour, but it did help Gary. More than that, it led to something which changed our lives.

Whilst I was waiting for Gary to finish a hyperbaric chamber session one day, I picked up two books in the waiting room: "*The Enzyme Factor*" by Dr Hiromi Shinya, and a book about "The Acid Alkaline Connection". This book was about the importance of getting your body alkaline. Just looking at the cover, something hit home with me. Something connected.

Two weeks later, we were flying home. By then I had read both books cover to cover. At the very same time, my brother Michael was flying from Calgary to Vancouver after a business trip. Whilst on the plane, he was sitting next to a Filipino man. They chatted a bit and exchanged business cards and when they got off the plane, Michael thought nothing more of it.

The next morning, I was having a casual chat with Michael and I told him what I had read in the book. I said that I was going out to find a water ionizer machine right away. There was a kind of stunned silence and then Michael said, "Hang on, what did you say?" I repeated it, and he said, "Suz, you are never gonna believe this..." Turns out, the Filipino business man, who he was sitting next to on the plane, sold the very machine I wanted to buy: his was 'the gold standard' of all water ionizers from Japan.

I started to get excited and said, "I have to have one of these machines! This is the missing link!" Gary was listening to me as I was talking to Michael, and as I put the phone down, he said wearily, "What the fuck are you talking about?"

I explained to Gary how we had to have a water machine. He scoffed. I think he swore at me again.

Michael told me to sit tight while he researched the machines. He called me back a few hours later, saying that he had looked into all the machines on the market and it seemed that the one I should buy was indeed the one that the Filipino man sold. I call this "divine intervention".

Gary had other ideas. He told me flat out I was not allowed to buy one. We had, after all, spent a lot of money trying to get Gary well; this was another expense we could do without.

I contacted the local distributor, Joe. I asked – I may have insisted – that he come over immediately to give us a demonstration. When Joe arrived, Gary was on the patio and wouldn't even come into the house. I demanded he come in, which he reluctantly did. About ten minutes into the demo, I told Joe I wanted a machine. Gary was furious. He said he was going to leave me. "Gary, I am saving your life here. We are buying this machine."

"No, we are not!" stormed Gary.

Of course, we bought the machine.

I was like Nurse Ratched after that. I would make sure Gary drank his allotted water every day, sometimes pouring it out and keeping watch until he'd drunk it. It was a struggle at first, but after a while it became a habit. Gary started to feel better, and after four weeks, his health had turned around and he was a different man.

Strangely enough, my health changed too, without me even trying. I had been so focused on getting Gary well, that I didn't even consider what it would do for me.

On Father's Day that year, our girls came to visit. A year before, these girls weren't sure their dad would see another Father's Day, so that was a special year for us. Not only was their dad still here, but he was happy and connected, and back to his old self.

In Robert G Wright's book, "*Killing Cancer - Not People*", he says: "Cancer, obesity, high blood pressure, diabetes, arthritis, kidney/renal disease, cardio-vascular disease, ad infinitum, are all slowed, stopped and in most circumstances reversed when drinking ionised water".

Acidity in the body promotes disease. It is essential that we limit the acidity that goes into our bodies. But most of the water we drink is actually acidic. We know how important water consumption is, so to maximise the benefits of water, it makes sense that we would consume alkaline water.

Dr Ray Kurzweil and Dr Terry Grossman, authors of "*Fantastic Voyage: Live Long Enough to Live Forever*" say: "Consuming the right type of water is vital to detoxifying the body's acidic waste products and is one of the most powerful health treatments available. We recommend that you drink 8-10 glasses per day of this alkaline water."

Dr Warburg was one of the Twentieth Century's leading cell biologists. He discovered that the root cause of cancer is too much acidity in the body, meaning that the pH – potential hydrogen – in the body is below the normal level of 7.365, which constitutes an "acidic" state. Dr Warburg investigated the metabolism of tumours and the respiration of cells and discovered that cancer cells maintain and thrive in a lower pH, as low as 6.0, due to lactic acid production and elevated CO_2. He firmly believed that there was a direct relationship between pH and oxygen. Higher pH, which is alkaline, means higher concentration of oxygen molecules, while lower pH, which is acidic, means lower concentrations of oxygen... the same oxygen that is needed to maintain healthy cells.

In 1931 he was awarded the Nobel Prize in medicine for this important discovery.

In his work "*The Metabolism of Tumours*", Dr Warburg demonstrated that all forms of cancer are characterized by two basic conditions: acidosis and hypoxia (lack of oxygen). "Lack of oxygen and acidosis are two sides of the same coin; where you have one, you have the other. All normal cells are an absolute requirement for oxygen, but cancer cells can live without oxygen – a rule without exception. Deprive a cell 35% of its oxygen for 48 hours and it may become cancerous."

Dr Warburg made it clear that the root cause of cancer is oxygen deficiency, which creates an acidic state in the human body. He also discovered that cancer cells are anaerobic (do not breathe oxygen) and cannot survive in the presence of high levels of oxygen, as found in an alkaline state.

Drinking ionized water has been essential in Gary's recovery, and I am certain it has also played a role in mine. We are both religious about drinking it every day, and I will do so for the rest of my life. In our case, there is definitely something in the water...

CHAPTER SEVEN

SHE WEARS MY RING

"Praise the bridge that carried you over."

—*George Colman the Younger*

In Gary's words

Our lives changed forever after Suzie was diagnosed with cancer. I did not, and still do not, understand it.

How could this happen to someone who was so much into health and nutrition? Suzie had always been a keen advocate of healthy eating, even when our girls were small; she instilled it into all of us how important our health was and how to protect it.

Every morning before I would get up, I would hear her grinding organic wheat to make flour so she could make her own bread. She would constantly juice, long before it was fashionable to do so. We ate a lot of plant based foods. Nutrition was a priority in our home.

We now know that even though we were eating healthily, we were drinking acidic waters; we didn't actually have a clue.

When Suzie's diagnosis came, I knew I would be there for her, no matter what. But I also knew that, even if I had chosen not to support her, she would do it her way, regardless. She is a strong-willed and determined person, and fighting cancer was just another battle for her – one that she was determined to win.

After the diagnosis came the pressure to have treatment. You get into the system when you have cancer, and it's hard to get out.

At Suzie's oncologist appointment in Vancouver, we were told that the doctors wanted to use an experimental chemo drug and Tamoxifen. I realised after about five minutes into the appointment that what we were being subjected to was a canned pitch. The oncologist started out by saying, "We are going to try chemo," as if it was unlikely that it would work.

The speech was well rehearsed, and not open for discussion or debate; though of course this oncologist was soon to get exactly that from Suzie. I started to wonder how many people blindly accept this patter, unquestioningly, and this upset me. In the world of oncology, there are few choices. But we all have choices and we all have the right to choose; Suzie taught me that. What we were being given was a death sentence, with no hope; no light; no alternatives.

Despite Suzie's protests, the nurses started to take blood from her arm (which we later found out was to see how compatible she was with this particular chemo), but as the needle was being inserted, my wife became angry and pulled the needle out of her arm. She said, "Let's get the hell out of here," and at that point I knew that she would be seeking an alternative treatment.

She had many sleepless nights, but I could see a determination and resolve in her. She absolutely believed that she would kick this cancer. She knew a lot about the body and health and she knew she had to get her immune system strong so it could fight the disease without chemo. There was never a doubt, not one, that she would choose the conventional route.

For the next few weeks she drove every day an hour each way, in rush hour traffic, to a naturopath clinic to get Vitamin C drips and antioxidant vitamins. She read countless books and researched alternative healing, until she came across the Gerson therapy in

Mexico. Once she told me about this place, I knew that's where we would be heading.

For three weeks in Mexico, I slept in a bed beside her; I watched many of the procedures; went to the lectures, assisted as much as I could. The coffee enemas presented a challenge for me – not only was I a little sceptical, but I was always a little concerned that they were wasting good coffee!

At the clinic, I ate the same kind of food she ate – no salt, no sugar, no additives, no butter, no bread. Even though I was used to eating a healthy diet, this was different. It took some getting used to. I can't deny that I would sneak out to get "normal" food when I could.

For those three weeks, Suzie's day from morning until night was long, tedious and draining. She was one of the few who came to the clinic without ever having undergone chemo; most came as a last resort after the chemo hadn't worked for them. Some of the patients were really, really sick, and it was tough to see. I honestly felt that Suzie was the only one who looked healthy. The more time I spent there, the more I started to believe that it would work; the more faith I had that she would beat this thing that had over-taken our lives.

She would say to me, "I never want to own this disease. I will never give it any power by saying 'I have cancer.'" What a positive and strong woman my wife is.

We learned so much during those three weeks. Suzie would take it all in and apply it to her recovery. It was a life changing journey that I will never forget, and I believe it saved her. Who knew that one day we would need this knowledge later in our lives, not just for my own illness, but for our youngest daughter.

In 2003, I was diagnosed with prostate cancer. Suzie was there to help me make some lifestyle changes, and she was also there to remind me not to have radiation or chemo. My doctor would con-stantly say to me, "You have got to do something about it!" and I would respond that I was doing something about it; just not what he was telling me to do. I knew I did not want to have my prostate removed; I had seen too many good friends now in diapers; some of whom even had the cancer return after the operation.

On one of the last visits to my doctor he said to me, "Your PSA is over 35 and if you don't do something about it, you will die." I replied, "I am doing something about it. I am changing my diet and lifestyle." And that's what I started to do.

But then in 2005, I was rushed to hospital with a terrible case of IBS colitis. I had five operations over a three month period. They removed most of my colon. I lost 70 pounds. They sent me home to die. I had PTSD, sleep apnea, hiatus hernia, heart arrhythmia, neuropathy and major congestion. I was continually nauseous. This all stemmed from the five operations I had had.

For two and a half years after these surgeries, I would sit in a corner of the living room waiting to die. Later I learned that my neighbours had nicknamed me "Dead Man Walking". Suzie kept me alive with Vitamin C drips, Myers cocktails (the best non alcoholic cocktail you can find!) and good, nutritious food.

And now it was my turn to go out of town for treatment. We made a trip to the Whittaker Wellness Centre in Newport Beach, in California. We spent two weeks there whilst I received heart treatments, Vitamin C, chelation and shock treatment therapy (for the neuropathy). We attended lectures on health. I started to improve, but I was far from feeling that sense of wellbeing that had been missing from my life. It was here on this trip that Suzie picked up a book about the acid / alkaline connection. And at this moment, I truly believe, our lives changed. After reading the book, Suzie was convinced that my body wasn't getting well because it was too acidic. In typical Suzie style, she told me we must buy an alkaline water machine. Immediately.

I wasn't convinced, and to be honest I resisted buying that machine. But Suzie is a force to be reckoned with, and the resistance was futile. The machine was ordered, installed and up and running within days of our return home from California.

Suzie made sure I drank half my body weight of alkaline water in ounces every day. It took around a month before I started to re-alise that I felt better. Not just better, but well. After another few weeks, I wasn't just well – but healthy. It was amazing.

I drink the alkaline water every day and I love it. I have not had a cold or flu or any sickness in that whole time. I believe that Suzie's determination saved my life.

Having been though, and witnessed, disease in our lives, I have come to a few realisations. I really believe that we have to try to eliminate stress from our lives; eat 80% plant-based, organic foods, and never drink soda or pop. We should drink ionized, alkaline mi-cro-clustered water; the same kind of water the Hunza* people in the Himalayas drink. Oh, and I believe that men should not have prostate biopsy, as this can cause the cancer to spread. I was told this by a prominent US doctor, and I believe it.

Over the years, I am glad to say I have learned a lot about health. God gave us these wonderful bodies and above all, we have amazing immune systems that have the ability to fight disease. We are all subjected to free radicals constantly invading our bodies, and we have to learn how to strengthen our immune systems so they can fight the free radicals and keep our bodies strong.

It's ten years on from my prostate cancer diagnosis, and I am still here. The love of my life is still here too. If I was to thank God, I would also have to thank Suzie. Between them, they've done a pretty good job.

*The Hunza people

The Story of the Hunza people is very interesting. For centuries, rumours of an earthly paradise hidden in an almost inaccessible valley in the high Himalayas in northern India intrigued the outside world with stories of a "lost race" who had learned to stop the ageing process.

Occasional travellers returned with incredible stories of a nation where people stayed youthfully active for as long as they lived and where "young" people of a hundred years or more were the rule instead of the exception.

The people of Hunza have evolved a way of living, eating and thinking that has substantially lengthened their lifespan and dramatically reduced susceptibility to most of the illnesses to which "civilised" people are prone.

In Hunza, people manage to live to over 100 years of age in perfect mental and physical health; and men can father children at 90. Cancer, heart disease, heart attacks, high and low blood pressure and childhood diseases are virtually unknown. In fact, sickness is extremely rare.

Dr Robert McCarrison, a brilliant English surgeon, took up the study of certain diseases common to the people of Asia. He was interested in finding out to what degree diseases in Indian peoples were caused by faulty food. He was amazed by the remarkable health and vitality of these people. He wrote in his classic book *"Studies in deficiency diseases"*:

"My own experience provides an example of a race unsurpassed in perfection of physique and in freedom from disease in general. I refer to the people of the State of Hunza, situated in the extreme northernmost point of India (now part of Pakistan). Amongst these people the span of life is extraordinarily long. During the period of my association with these people, I never saw a case of asthenic dyspepsia, of gastric or duodenal ulcer, or appendicitis, or mucous colitis, or cancer."

Dr McCarrison proceeded to view the ills of both civilised and primitive man. The only difference he could find was in their diet. The Hunzas practised a spartan form of agriculture, returning all organic matter to the soil. Their food consisted chiefly of raw fruits and vegetables, sprouted pulses, whole grains, nuts milk products from goats, and occasionally a small portion of meat, usually during holidays and weddings. Since chickens have a natural urge to peck at seeds, and since seeds are more valuable than money in Hunza, until recently no chickens were allowed in the state.

Very little fat of any kind is consumed by the people through ghee, butter apricot oil and negligible quantities of animal fats.

Most foods are consumed raw. There is a complete absence of foreign additives; nothing whatsoever is added to either the soil or the food of the people or the animals. No sprays or spray materials of any kind are used on their crops, and no unnatural chemical fertilisers are used on their lands. All fruits and vegetables that are dried for storing have been exposed to the sun and air.

Nobel Prize winner Dr. Henri Coanda spent six decades studying the Hunza water trying to determine what it was in their water that caused such beneficial effects for the body. He discovered that it had a different viscosity and surface tension. Dr. Patrick Flanagan and others continued the research. They found Hunza water had a high alkaline pH and an extraordinary amount of active hydrogen (hydrogen with an extra electron), with a negative Redox Potential and a high colloidal mineral content. The water is living and provides health benefits that other types of drinking water cannot. Similar natural water properties and longevity are found in other remote unpolluted places such as the Shin-Chan areas of China, the Caucasus in Azerbaijan, and in the Andes Mountains.

This article about Gary appeared in the Peace Arch News newspaper in 2009. It was written by Juliet Sullivan.

Big Gary is big. He is a man with presence, an awe-inspiring energy, and a story to tell. He is tall, strong, and healthy. But it wasn't always that way. In fact, just a short time ago, Big Gary was not so big, and certainly not so healthy. He had undergone a series of operations, had lost 70 pounds, and was lying in a hospital bed, close to death.

Gary Derrett is a well-known figure in South Surrey. Up until three years ago, he owned and ran a chain of vacuum stores throughout the Lower Mainland: "Big Gary's." He did this for more than 40 years.

Gary was not a healthy man. He had suffered 20 years of colitis and Irritable Bowel Syndrome (IBS). He had learned to live with, and tolerate, the illnesses, as many people do.

And then one day, 3½ years ago, he was rushed to emergency with severe swelling to his stomach. He was on the operating table for six hours, after his colon burst and he almost died.

After the operation, his stomach became infected, a staph infection so bad that he underwent five further surgeries over the course of three months. The infection went on for half a year.

"They used a vise and staples to keep me together," says Gary. "And – ironically – a vacuum to clean me out. I don't think it was one of mine though."

The household-appliance entrepreneur can joke about it now, but at the time, the pain was so intense that Gary says he had never known what real pain was until that time. Nurses have since told him they had never seen a patient administered so much morphine.

Before the fifth operation, hospital staff advised Gary's family to gather around him, with doctors suggesting it was unlikely he would come out of the surgery alive.

Against the odds, he did come out alive, but that was just the beginning. There was a long and painful road ahead. "Basically, they sent Gary home to die," says wife Suzie.

Once home, Gary started to suffer depression, anxiety, headaches, nausea, chronic fatigue, major arthritis, sleep apnea and lung congestion He had post traumatic stress and had to walk with the aide of a walker. Neighbours have since told him that they gave him a nickname in those days: "Dead Man Walking." It got worse.

In April 2008, Gary was driving home one day and started to suffer heart palpitations. After tests, his doctor told him his heart was damaged and enlarged, and he had developed heart arrhythmia (irregular heartbeat), sometimes so bad that Gary thought he was having a heart attack.

Some time after that, Suzie received a newsletter from a wellness centre in Newport Beach, California. In it, they talked about heart arrhythmia and how they could cure it with magnesium.

"Suzie had me on a plane down there the very next day – in a wheelchair," says Gary.

The wellness centre treated Gary with a series of natural remedies. Two weeks – and $25,000 – later, Gary says the heart arrhythmia subsided and he felt "a little better," even though the centre had diagnosed yet another problem: neuropathy (numbness) in his feet and legs.

"I was waiting for some kind of magic, but it never came. Basically, I felt like I was on my way out. I felt like it was the end. I even contacted my life insurance provider, just to make sure that everything was in order..."

And then, on the flight back home, Suzie read a book. The book was about balancing the PH in the body, and talked about how disease thrives in an acidic body; something most of us, unfortu-nately, possess.

Due to bad eating habits, smoking, lifestyle and environmental toxins, the level of PH in most of our bodies is unbalanced. This is making us sick, fat and tired. It claimed that by increasing the al-kalinity in the body, simply by drinking alkaline water, disease will no longer be able to flourish.

"I read this book and it made so much sense," Suzie says. "I felt that it was the missing link in Gary's health."

Suzie knew she had to find a way to make Gary's body more alka-line. Unfortunately, alkaline water machines are not exactly com-mon here. Widely used in Japanese hospitals for decades, the technology has only recently come to North America, and there is still a certain skepticism surrounding their effectiveness.

But when you are the proactive, forward-thinking wife of a de-pressed, dying man to whom you have been married for 43 years, you will ignore skepticism and employ your own judgement. Suzie was willing to try anything to help her beloved Gary. And here is where fate stepped in.

As Suzie and Gary were flying back from Newport Beach, Suzie's brother Michael was on a plane flying back from Calgary. He sat next to a man on the flight, whose business happened to be alka-line water machines.

Despite Gary's doubts, they bought a machine. Gary started to drink alkaline water. Six glasses a day at first, gradually building up until Gary says his body was craving it.

Fast forward 3½ weeks. Father's Day 2008. Gary's four daughters wanted to take a family portrait on the beach, complete with 11 grandchildren.

"My girls thought it was my last Father's Day," says Gary, tearfully. "On the day before the photo shoot, Suzie had asked me to make sure it was a good day; in other words that I fake it. I still didn't have that sense of wellbeing and she knew I could be difficult sometimes.

"But that morning, I noticed when I woke up that I didn't have the usual nausea, or aches. Instead of taking an hour to get out of bed, get dressed and go downstairs, as I had done for the past three years, it took me five minutes. I felt good, but I kept thinking it wouldn't last.

"Later that day, after lunch, I got up from the table and went to each of my daughters and grandchildren, kissed them and told them I loved them. It was like I was reborn. I had that sense of wellbeing back that was robbed from me for over three years.

"Later, back home, Suzie said to me, 'Thank you for making an effort today.' And I looked at her and said 'I got news for you – I feel good!' All day I had been expecting the walls to come crashing down, but they never did."

And they still haven't. Ten months later, Gary feels more alive, more energized, and more healthy than ever.

He is back playing golf. He walks. ("I walk like I'm on a marathon," he says). He is full of life. His energy is contagious. His neuropathy has totally vanished, as has his heart arrhythmia. Doctors had told him that he would have both these conditions for the rest of his life.

There is, however, one condition his family has noticed with all this improved health. "He didn't really talk for three years," Suzie says. "Now he won't shut up!"

Big Gary is a man with a mission, and a story to tell.

CHAPTER EIGHT
You'll Never Walk Alone

"Experience is the worst teacher. It always gives the test first and the instruction afterward."

—*Niklaus Wirth*

In the summer of 2010, my youngest daughter Shannon came to me with the words that no mother ever wants to hear. "Mom, I have breast cancer." Excuse me for swearing, but FUCK! Will this disease never leave my family alone? Anger out of the way, I went into warrior mode. We would just have to fight another battle, that's all.

Though I was sad, I was never scared for her. I knew that this was just another test; something we would come through together. On that awful day when she was diagnosed, she was understandably distraught. She was crying hysterically in my arms and told me that the doctor told her she must go to see the oncologist.

But I had other ideas. I did not want her to go to see any oncologists. I knew they would scare her. They may even scare her into having chemotherapy. I had total faith in treating it naturally, and that's not easy for a mother to say. Making that kind of decision for myself – easy. It's my life, my body. Making that decision for my daughter? Without absolute faith and belief – impossible. *With* absolute faith and belief – it's what they call a 'no brainer'.

Shannon's was an aggressive cancer and there seemed little option but to undergo a double mastectomy. Some weeks later, as I watched my baby girl being wheeled away for the operation, I said, "Trouper, you are going to war, so get those army boots on!"

She raised her right arm, smiled weakly, and gave a salute.

And I thought, "She's on a journey, my girl." It's not a journey I would have chosen for her, but I accepted it, as I had accepted my own journey, and my mother's before us.

After the operation, and during Shannon's recovery, the doctor told Shannon's husband Steve that it was imperative that she goes to the Cancer Clinic; they said that due to the aggressiveness of the cancer, chemo was absolutely necessary.

Shannon had already started the Gerson at that point. She was following it religiously at home and was committed to a fully natural recovery. I asked Shannon, "If you go to see an oncologist, whatever they tell you, what would you do differently?"

She replied, "Nothing." So, my point was: what was the point?

She never saw an oncologist.

That's my girl.

In Shannon's words

"You never know how strong you are until being strong is the only choice you have!"

—*Unknown*

When my mom was diagnosed with breast cancer, I remember thinking "Cancer equals death." I felt powerless and hopeless. I knew nothing about the disease, and I guess ignorance equals fear.

I begged her to have chemo, as at the time I knew a girl my age who had breast cancer and was going through the treatments; she seemed to be doing OK – well, apart from the hair loss, extreme fatigue, and sallow complexion.

In response to this, my mom said, "There is no way I will poison myself," and I was confused. Chemo is supposed to make you well. How can it be poison? But when I look back at what my friend was going through, that is exactly what was happening to her – she was being poisoned.

After a while, I relaxed. My mom made having cancer look easy. In truth, I don't think I ever really knew how devastating it was for her and my dad. They just got on with it, and us girls never really knew the struggles they were facing. My mom listened to Elvis a lot, and he seemed to bring her strength and calm. I am grateful that he was there for her.

I actually remember being at the hospital on the evening of her mastectomy, looking at my mom as she listened to music on her CD player, and thinking: "It's OK. Elvis has got this!"

When she returned from her time at the Gerson in Mexico, she was constantly juicing. She spent a lot of time in the bathroom doing coffee enemas and that was one thing I really didn't understand.

But as that year went by, my fear of losing her subsided. She amazed me, and still does, with her courage, strength and determination. I had no idea that, 16 years later, I would need some of that courage and strength myself.

It was July 1st 2010 when I found a lump in my right breast. It's hard to explain the fear that descends upon you when you find a lump. It's kind of like a lingering wave that is washing over you, drowning your sense of peace and well-being. You don't yet know what it is, but it's still scary. I had an ultrasound. The results said it was "Fibroadenoma" (non-cancerous breast lumps).

I was then referred to a surgeon, who read the report, examined me and concluded, "It's not breast cancer because it's painful when touched." Cancer doesn't hurt, he said. He told me to go away and enjoy my summer.

I was told to return on September 24th so he could remove the lump. But I didn't really enjoy my summer. I knew something wasn't right. And then another lump appeared.

When I went back to the surgeon in September for the lumpectomy, I told him about the second lump. I told him it felt like octopus tentacles. That day, both lumps were removed and the surgeon told me he would get his secretary to call me when the pathology report was back.

Five days later, I got the call from the secretary, and I was back in his office pretty quickly after that. Relieved that the lumps were gone, I walked in and said cheerily, "Wow, you did a nice job on my breast." He was quiet. I thought he looked a little upset. My heart started to race.

"You have breast cancer," he said.

I felt like I was going to pass out. Everything you think you know about yourself disappears in a moment like that. You think you might be hysterical, dramatic... and you're calm, composed. The surgeon said, "I am so sorry," but I hugged him and said, "It's OK."

That night, I tried to sleep but found my thoughts drifting to a place of pure fear. I was at my own funeral; I could see my three beautiful children crying and my husband holding on to them. Then I saw my mom and dad in pain. I had to stop myself from thinking these dark thoughts. I lay awake all night, and many more nights after that.

The doctors recommended a double mastectomy, and I agreed. I wanted that cancer out of me.

One day sometime before the surgery, my mom had a spiritual healer come to her house to see me. Mom told me not to tell her anything about myself, so I didn't. As I lay down on the bed, she told me she will be placing her hands above my whole body, but will not be touching me. She told me to close my eyes and then she took me on a guided visual experience that blew my mind.

She determined that I had a blockage - something in my past I couldn't seem to let go and forgive myself for. She was right. All I can say is, she helped me let go that day. After my session, she told me to open my eyes and she said, "Shannon, you have breast cancer; it's in your right breast." I had not told her this. I was amazed.

She explained to me that breast cancer on the right side represented resentment and anger. I remembered a book I once read that stated "most diseases have an emotional root."

One night, a few days before the operation, in the middle of the night, I felt the presence of my dear Grandma Val beside me. She put her hand on my head and whispered, "Everything will be OK, dear." I really didn't think I was dreaming, because I had never experienced anything like it before.

In the morning, I told my mom about the experience with Grandma Val, and she said, "Was it at around 3am?" I said, "Yes," and she said, "She came to me also." We both cried.

Just before my surgery, during another phone call to my mom, she could sense that I was still full of fear. She snapped, "This is enough! No more giving fear anymore power! I will let you have one more week of fear, and then no more!" I have to admit, she did snap me out of it.

The night before the op, I lay on my bed crying. I was so scared to have both breasts removed. It felt so final and so radical. My two boys came in to the bedroom and lay with me. I cried to them, "I don't want to have this surgery." But I could see how scared they both were, as they held me. They asked me to do it, for them.

On the day of the surgery, husband Steve – and my new friend Ativan - helped me get to the hospital for 6am. I had a support group waiting for me – family and friends – and they watched as I was wheeled down the hallway, my mom calling out, "Get your army boots on – you are going to war!" I raised my arm in salute, and I even think I raised a smile.

Of course, the next thing I knew I was laying in the recovery room, minus my breasts. It was a humbling, terrifying experience, and I knew I still had a long road ahead.

When I met my surgeon to go over the pathology report, I learned that there had been three tumours, measuring 8.5 centimetres. It was graded as Stage IIIB. A 1cm tumour contains on average one billion cells. Mine was 8.5cm. That's eight and a half billion cells!

They had also taken two lymph nodes, one of which did have signs of cancer in it. The surgeon said he would like to remove more lymph nodes, to be sure. "No way," I said.

I asked if I would need chemo. He nodded gravely and said, "Yes, we have an oncologist's number for you to call."

My reply was this: "I would rather die than do chemo."

He was absolutely shocked; speechless in fact.

At the hospital a few days later for a follow-up appointment, my mom started talking to my surgeon about a hormone pill that I had been taking before I found the lump. This hormone pill had been prescribed to me by a doctor in Vancouver, who had put me on 50mg of DHEA, which I had been taking faithfully for seven months. The surgeon asked for the doctor's name and then he pulled a medical book from his shelf and started looking through it. He found what he was looking for, and then said, "This doctor is not even a hormone specialist!"

I asked him if the DHEA could have caused the tumours; he said he thought it was possible as the third tumour was growing so fast and down to the chest wall.

He also said that the implants I had in my chest saved my life, because they stopped the tumours going into my lungs.

My subsequent research on DHEA in high doses shows that it affects the estrogen in your body and turns it into bad estrogen.

When given HRT it is important to get your hormone levels checked every two to three months, which in my case was never done. Also, when you have a history of breast cancer in your family, never take high doses of DHEA.

I wish I had known then what I know now. There are risks of taking high doses of DHEA which was never explained to me. I felt – and still feel – so much anger towards that "doctor".

Ten months later I decided to confront her; I needed to forgive. I don't believe in carrying anger and resentment around with me. I told her, "All I want you to know for future clients, is to please check their DHEA levels when you put them on such a high dose, and to supplement them with Indole-3-Carbinol." I felt like I was the doctor.

She did seem genuinely sorry – she knew she was wrong; she asked to hug me. As I left, she said, "Shannon, you are an honourable woman." I really did not know what that meant. I still don't. I just don't want other women to go through a similar experience.

And so began my recovery. After spending two weeks at my parents' house, I went home to start the Gerson therapy in full. It was, to put it mildly, not an easy time. Basically, my day consisted of regular juicing, coffee enemas, Vitamin B12 injections, and other treatments. It was a strict regime that took over my life for three months. But it also saved my life.

At that time, I was referred to a Gerson trained doctor who practiced in Kirkland, Washington. I would fax all my reports and blood tests to her over that whole year and we would have phone consultations. This woman is so knowledgeable and I learned a lot about health from her. I have never met her, and one day would love to tell her she was an angel sent to me. This woman has been a big part of my recovery.

I found that my own medical doctor was not supportive of my choices and I decided I needed to find a new one. My mother in law told me about her own female doctor; a progressive visionary who did not seem bound by convention. She agreed to take me on and throughout all of this has been incredibly supportive.

The spiritual healer who had told me that I had breast cancer just before my operation, came back to my house a few weeks after the mastectomy. At the end of our session, she said to me, "Shannon, the cancer has gone." These are some of the best words I have ever heard in my life.

One year after the first diagnosis, I had a CT scan which confirmed the healer's words: I was cancer free. As my new medical doctor gave me the results of the scan, she hugged me and said, "Keep doing what you're doing, Shannon."

I celebrated that day. First with a beautiful, healthy lunch with my mom... and then at the tattoo parlour, where I got a tattoo on my wrist with the word: "Survivor".

Deciding to have reconstruction surgery was not easy, but I am young and I want to feel like a woman, and so I opted to have implants a year after my mastectomy.

Seven months after surgery, I had tissue expanders put in. I wore them for six long and painful months. They were hard and uncomfortable, especially at bedtime. I had to have saline injections every two to three weeks. I remember my friend Juliet coming with me to my doctor's appointment and holding my hand. I think I may have cut her with my nails from squeezing so tight.

During that time, I experienced these really bizarre episodes where my legs – from my hips to my shins - would ache so badly that I was hospitalized three times. I later had an intravenous heavy metal test and discovered that I had high levels of mercury and other heavy metals in my body.

My battles were clearly not just with cancer.

Almost six months after having the tissue expanders put in, I called the surgeon's secretary to tell her about my heavy metal test and that I wanted these expanders out as soon as possible. She was always so kind and nice to me; and this day she heard the concern in my voice; she called me back right away with good news that I could get them out within two weeks.

After I had them removed, I did not get any more awful leg pains. I believe that those excruciating pains were a result of my body rejecting the metal portal inside the tissue expanders. Once they were gone, so was the pain.

After my final surgery on December 1st 2011, I was so happy that it was all over that within ten days I was dancing at my husband's Christmas party.

That year, on New Year's Eve, on our 15th wedding anniversary, Steve and I renewed our vows. We did it at Juliet's house, surrounded by our dear friends and family. The ceremony was presided over by someone who is very special to me – Reverend Terry; a man who has helped me so many ways throughout my journey, not only with my breast cancer but in life.

The renewing of the vows was a surprise for husband Steve.

When we arrived, my mom and dad and Steve's parents and some friends were in the bedroom (because seeing them downstairs would have given it away to Steve).

So I quickly put on my dress (the same one I wore on my wedding day), and I walked downstairs to "*The one I love*" by David Gray. My dad walked me down the stairs into the family room and Steve was truly surprised.

I looked around the room at all my friends and family and thought to myself, "These are the people who have been here with me from the start." I was emotional, yet happy at the same time. I will never forget how special that night was for me.

Recently, my best friend (another Shannon) gave me a book called, "*Hello Susan It's me Cancer,*" by Susan D'Agostino. She had read the back of the book and saw that the author had treated her cancer naturally; she knew this book would interest me. I started reading it a couple of days later and there was a chapter called "*A friend of a friend's mother."* In the chapter, Susan credited this woman (the friend of a friend's mother) with helping to save her life.

As I started reading it, I got goose bumps. Her account of what the friend's friend's mom (all of whom were un-named in the book) had told her sounded so much like my mom that it was almost surreal. I became convinced that this was my mom she was writing about. So the next morning, I looked up the number for the author and I called her. And she confirmed: yes, it was indeed my mom! I, of course, am the friend's friend, but I still don't know who our mutual friend is.

It was amazing to speak to someone my mom helped. Not only that, but this lady was still alive and coming up to her 8 year celebration of being cancer free.

The chapter is shown below, with kind permission of the author:

My Friend's Friend's Mom
A Little Bird Told me

I was on a roller coaster of emotions. I wanted to believe there was a natural way to heal from this dis-ease, but I did not know anyone with knowledge of how to begin or what to do. I had only a few weeks until I was supposed to start chemotherapy. My mind was racing most days. I did not know where to begin and I was stressed out, exhausted and emotional. I felt I was waiting to get sick, or maybe waiting to die. It just didn't make any sense to me to kill off my immune system. What made sense to me was to build up my immune system. But I didn't know how to do that on my own. On a good day, when I considered following the natural way, I felt really good and I had lots of energy. I went for long walks in the forest with my dog. On a bad day, when I didn't feel so good, I felt depressed, hopeless, and thought maybe it was my time to die.

Some days I stayed in my pajamas all day; some days I stayed in bed all day.

On a warm Saturday, August 20th, I opted to stay in bed all day; I didn't see a purpose in getting up. A friend telephoned me at 2.30 in the afternoon and asked how I was doing. I was crying and watching TV in bed. She once again told me of her friend's mother who did natural treatments and wondered, if she got the telephone number, would I call her friend's mom? I told her the lady would think it was a prank call because I could not speak without crying, my voice would tighten up, and sometimes no words came out or else my voice sounded very high and squeaky. She said she would call the lady and have her friend's mom call me. I agreed to that arrangement. After I hung up the telephone, I felt a huge surge of energy fill my body. There was hope! I threw my blanket off and I ran into the bathroom to have a shower. I was so excited and energized – suddenly I felt so good.

When the phone rang a while later it was her. I explained to her where I was in the process, that I had had surgery and a partial mastectomy, and she began to speak very passionately about what I needed to do. I told her I smoked a little and I thought she was going to come right through the telephone at me! She told me, very loudly, that I couldn't do both! She told me to just stop it; that smoking cigarettes robs the body of oxygen! Either I keep smoking and do conventional treatments or I don't take one more puff and no natural treatments. She told me about some treatments – coffee enemas, intravenous vitamin C, and drinking freshly squeezed juices – which cleanse the body. She knew of a naturopath who maybe could help me. She told me about an integrated healing clinic in the city, explained that cancer hates oxygen, so exercise is good. She also suggested letting go of the fear since cancer feeds on fear. Stop eating sugar and stop drinking alcohol.

She said to take one day at a time and get a passion for life. I honestly didn't have a clue about how to get a passion for life. She directed me to go to the beach and give everything I didn't want back to the universe. She asked me what I could do today. I thought that maybe I could go to the organic vegetable farm to get some vegetables to juice.

She shared very little about her story. She had gone to Mexico for natural treatments eight years previous. At that time, the doctors here had given her only months to live. I have never met this lady in person, but I am eternally grateful for her passion and for helping me to save my life. I have never had another cigarette.

After that telephone conversation, I went to the organic farm for some fresh vegetables to juice. Whenever my friends and I walked on the beach we spent time thinking about what we wanted to give back to the universe. We would throw a rock into the ocean as a symbol for everything we wanted to give back. Then we would throw a rock and ask for what we wanted. We threw many rocks into the ocean that summer.

"Hello Susan, it's me – cancer", by Susan D'Agostino

These days, I have my sense of wellbeing back. Through hard work and determination, I have my health – and positivity – back. I feel fantastic, healthy and strong. I now know this nightmare called cancer was actually a gift...a gift to make me appreciate every day - and when I say this - with tears in my eyes - I mean and feel it.

My husband has been amazing, and without him – and without my mom – and the love and support of my incredible family and friends – my experience of cancer would have been a much more difficult one. It may have looked like I was holding it together some days, but inside I was often a mess. It was with the support of those around me that I managed to pull through, physically and mentally. Those people have left footprints in my heart.

From this long and painful journey, I have discovered that I want to give back and help others...just like my passionate mom...

"I see with love, dissolving all anger and resentment. Forgiveness dissolves all lingering toxic conditions in my body."

—Louise Hay

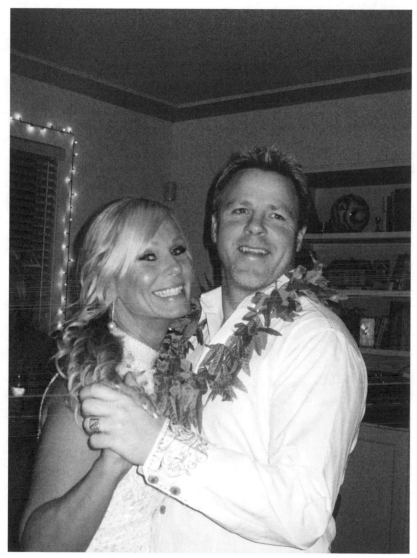

Steve and I when we renewed our vows

CHAPTER NINE
IT'S NOW OR NEVER

"Feeding your body chemicals is like putting sugar in the gas tank of your Maserati; that's the end of the car."

—Suzanne Somers

Shannon's tips for living a healthy life:

Not everybody can do The Gerson therapy, I know that. But everyone can change the way they eat. We should all be aware of what we are putting into our bodies.

After my extensive research, I now know that there are some foods that I absolutely will not put into my body, some I eat in moderation and some I can't get enough of. The following is my advice, based on what I have learned over the past few years.

I would recommend to anyone who has just been diagnosed with cancer, or anyone trying to live clean, that they say goodbye to the following:

- All meats and dairy

- Sugar

- Artificial sweeteners (poison!)

- Alcohol

- Canola oil

- Carageen (it's found in many nut milks)

- Table salt

- Gluten

- And Say NO to GMO's!

I would tell them to eat only organic produce, drink lots of alkaline water, make a green drink (recipe below) in a blender (that way all the goodness is not removed) and to juice carrot and apple every day.

They should eat a plant based diet, which includes hemp, chia, flax seeds, nuts, avocado, quinoa, Brussels sprouts, garlic, pineapple, cilantro etc.

Other tips:

- First thing in the morning, squeeze one organic lemon into warm water with a pinch of cayenne pepper. Very cleansing.

- Take a probiotic – for the rest of your life

- Take Chlorella (it will detoxify mercury from the body)

- Make sure your B-12 levels are in range (I get shots every month)

- Use Apple cider vinegar for salad dressings

- Consider having organic coffee enemas (I occasionally still do them)

- Take pancreatic enzymes after meals and before bed (it breaks down tumour tissue)

- Take liquid milk thistle in your water

- Take Vitamin D everyday (maybe back off a little in the hot summer months.)

EXERCISE! It will help drain your lymphatic system and help rid your body of waste. It also increases oxygen levels in the body, and cancer can't grow in high oxygen.

I also believe in Vitamin C drips. When I was first diagnosed, I would go three times a week. I still have them, as well as Vitamin K drips – Vitamin K is a great cancer fighting vitamin.

I also occasionally still have Myers cocktails – these are great for B12 and for the adrenal glands and stress.

Once in a while I try and kill candida in my body with Oil of Oregano capsules and liquid P'darco. I take both for a month. Before you start it, you spit in a glass of water first thing in the morning (before eating); if your spit drops to the bottom (like a tornado), it's time to kill those critters! I believe cancer is like a fungus.

Once a cancer sufferer is in the clear, they can adapt their diet and bring back certain foods in moderation. They can go out for a nice dinner but must still try to order clean. I still, to this day, change everything on a menu to suit myself - I'm paying for it after all. If the restaurant won't accommodate you, find a different restaurant.

- If you like wine, try stick to organic, and drink only occasionally.

- Wild salmon and halibut can be eaten but I always watch the amounts because I am concerned about mercury levels in our fish.

- If having coffee, make sure it's organic, not too frequent, and use almond milk, and grade 3 maple syrup as a sweetener.

- If you are a cheese lover, like me, you can eat organic white cheese occasionally. I try to stick to organic goat cheese as it's better for you.

"All disease begins in the gut."

—Hippocrates, the father of modern medicine

As a guide, you can replace the following bad guys with these good guys:

- Replace meat and dairy with quinoa/beans

- Replace refined sugar with raw unpasteurized honey

- Replace artificial sweeteners with Grade 3 Maple syrup

- Replace alcohol with Komucha fermented drinks

- Replace Canola oil with Coconut oil

- Replace table salt with Himalayan sea salt

- Replace gluten with coconut/brown rice/quinoa

- Replace fluoride toothpaste with a natural non-fluoride one

- Replace soap bars with natural peppermint soap or liquid

- Replace tap/bottled water with alkaline water

- Use natural deodorants and soaps

- Chlorine: purchase a shower head that will take out the chlorine in your water

- Replace body lotion with unrefined Shea butter or coconut oil

- Shampoo/conditioners - health food stores have many that are free of Phthalates and Sodium Lauryl Sulfate

• As for supplements, I take Co Q10, (UBIQUINOL), Selenium, zinc picolinate and a really good Vitamin C powder

• I also had Glutathione injections for the first year after being diagnosed, to repair my liver

I would like to share a few of my recipes with you; these are recipes that I have developed myself based on my own research, trial and error, and by using my family as guinea pigs. They are very happy, healthy guinea pigs though...

Spinach Pesto Quinoa Spaghetti

Ingredients

2 boxes of quinoa spaghetti (or brown rice spaghetti)

1 green onion chopped

1 red pepper chopped

1 red onion chopped

3 green onions - chopped

1 cup mushrooms - chopped (optional)

3 tbsp pesto

5 garlic cloves

2 cups washed spinach

1 package of small cherry tomatoes - sliced in half

¼ cup chopped basil

1 tsp coconut oil

Method

Saute 1 tsp coconut oil

Add all the veggies except spinach and cherry tomatoes

Once the vegetables are cooked (make sure not to overcook), add spinach and tomatoes, toss and cover with lid for 10 mins on a very low temperature.

Fill large pot with water and boil; place noodles in and stir occasionally - noodles will take longer than regular ones

Garnish with chopped fresh basil on top and a pinch of Himalayan sea salt

Chia pudding

Ingredients

    2/3 cup chia seeds

    1 tsp cinnamon

    2 cups true almond milk - unsweetened vanilla

    ½ tsp pure vanilla extract

    2 tbsp organic maple syrup

    2 tbsp unsweetened coconut flakes

Method

Put chia seeds, almond milk, coconut and vanilla in a 1 quart glass jar with a lid. Tighten the lid and shake well to thoroughly combine. Refrigerate overnight.

When ready to serve, stir well. Spoon into bowls and top with fruit.

Chia seeds soaked overnight turn into a simple pudding, similar in consistency to tapioca.

*Unsweetened almond milk contains only 30 calories per cup and is loaded with vitamins, minerals and antioxidants.

My green Alkalizing drink

I really enjoy this as my lunch some days. If I have eaten lunch, I make this around 3pm as a snack, and just omit the 2 scoops of vegan protein powder.

Ingredients

½ cup organic pineapple coconut juice

½ alkaline water

1 tbsp flax or Udo's oil

¼ cup blueberries

¼ of a banana

3 dandelion leaves

1 cup spinach

2 leaves collard greens

2 scoops of a Vegan protein powder

Method

Blend all ingredients well in blender

You can find more cancer fighting and preventing recipes in my cookbook:

Army * Strong
(My natural battle with cancer)
Healing recipes after the Gerson Therapy

www.recipesaftercancer.com

"The food you eat can either be the safest and most powerful form of medicine or the slowest form of poison."

Ann Wigmore

CHAPTER TEN
MY WAY

"All things must change to something new."

—Henry Wadsworth Longfellow

I don't know to this day how I did it, but I did. I had never known anyone who had done it my way, and have never met anyone since, apart from my daughter. That is a testament to how much I believe in it. To "fool around" with my own life – that's up to me. To recommend my daughter do the same – that was a test. But I believed it wholeheartedly. And I still do.

So, three generations of women in my family have had breast cancer; my mom, myself and Shannon. Having four grand-daughters, I decided it was a good idea to get genetic testing. If breast cancer was a genetic issue, those grand-daughters would have some important decisions to make.

Shannon's daughter, Krisdee, Shannon and myself all went for the tests. At the preliminary meeting, we were sitting with the doctor, talking about the history of cancer in our family. The doctor was taking notes and asking about my mother. "What treatment did she have?" she asked me.

I replied, "Nothing. They did offer cobalt treatment, which was all that was available back then, but she didn't take it."

"OK," she said, writing in her notes. "And what treatment did you have?" she asked me.

I replied, "Nothing."

"Nothing?"

"Well, I went to the Gerson in Mexico, but nothing conventional," I said.

She kept writing, in silence, her head down. "Obviously you took Tomoxifen?" she asked eventually. I could hear the strain in her voice.

"Nope."

There was more silence.

The doctor looked at my daughter and smiled, a touch nervously I thought...because I think she already knew the answer to her question: "So, Shannon, what treatment did you have?"

"Nothing," replied Shannon. By now, the doctor's eye was twitching. She looked like she was in pain, or at the very least distress. Was it my imagination or did her face go white?

Shannon and I laughed about it afterwards. But I was a little angry, because the doctor didn't ask us anything about what treatment we did employ. I wanted her to ask us, "Well what *have* you done? What *have* you changed in your life?"

As it turned out, that doctor is none the wiser about the two women sitting in her office that day, both of whom had beaten breast cancer without a single dose of conventional treatment. That level of narrow mindedness is a little disconcerting, don't you agree?

That day, on the way to the appointment, Krisdee and I got off on the wrong floor at the hospital, and there was an acrid burning smell in the halls. "Ugh..what is that smell? Is something burning?" Krisdee asked me.

"No, that's what cancer smells like," I replied. It was the smell of radiation and chemotherapy.

After our meeting with the doctor, the three of us stood in the middle of the hospital and hugged, thankful that we had not chosen to go down that poisonous road. We said a prayer for all those undergoing treatments, and felt blessed to have the knowledge and belief to know what we know about cancer.

Whether we choose the conventional or alternative road, I feel that cancer can be a lonely place, and we all need people to guide us, to help us through it.

Robert G Wright wrote in his book, "*Killing Cancer – Not People*":

What you must do first, though, what you must do right now, is to find an "advocate" - someone who will get onboard this train with you and ride in the seat right next to yours, holding your hand and guiding and supporting you on this journey. Without an advocate, you are traversing the 'minefield' of cancer therapies alone. And battling this disease by yourself can be frustrating, irritating, emotionally draining, and as a result, often ends tragically. So find a friend, a family member, a group, anyone who will sign-on to march lock step with you in your quest for healing, until you are well. Do it right away. I would make an 'advocate' one of my top priorities.

The first person who ever came to me for advice was a lady with breast cancer who had been sent to me by a neighbour. It was around a year after I returned from the Gerson. This lady was around 45. She knocked on my door one morning, holding a coffee, a box of doughnuts and a cigarette.

I answered the door, took one look at her and said, "You're not bringing any of that into my house." She reluctantly left her goodies outside, came in and I talked to her for a couple of hours about her need to make lifestyle changes. She sat and listened, and at the end of it she said, "I am not living like that. I can't give any of it up." She picked up her goodies and left. Six months later, my neighbour told me she had died.

Now, that lady may have died anyway – but she didn't give herself a chance to ever know any different; had she had made different choices, would she have lived another year, another ten years?

I am not claiming that I know best. I only know what I know. I know that if you change the terrain of your body, disease has a hard time being present in it. I know that what worked for me, and for my daughter.

I want more than anything to help people. I am telling my story in the hope that I can I do just that. Anyone who has cancer needs an advocate; someone who will support and understand their journey.

Robert G Wright also wrote in his book "*Killing Cancer - Not People*":

Always remember – don't panic – you almost always have time. Get your protocol together, do your homework, question all medical advice (question all advice – no matter where it comes from – question my advice, and check it out). Stop doing things that promote your cancer – start doing the things that will lead you to healing. That's what I would do.

Tomorrow is promised to no-one. We cannot choose how we are going to die, only how we are going to live. I choose to live each day to its fullest.

People ask me what got me through this time in my life. There are many things.

I believe that we all have to have a dream. At 67, I have done so much in my life, but I still have dreams and goals. My dearest **wish** is to see my girls, and my grandchildren, live strong, healthy lives. My biggest **dream** is to go to Graceland, home of Elvis.

I believe that we should live in faith, not fear. I myself believe in a higher power, whatever that is. Something bigger than myself. It worked for me. I don't follow a religion. I am a spiritual being having a human experience. I start my day and end my day by thanking "God" for the fact that I am here. Every day is a blessing to me.

Focus on why you want to stay around – for me it was my grandchildren.

From prolific reading, my own trial and error and experience, and from speaking with other people, this is what I believe in, for prevention and cure of cancer:

- Juice every day – it doesn't have to be 13 a day! I did 13 a day to start with, but nowadays I do one or two a day.

- Coffee enemas - to clean your liver. I know it sounds kooky, but I believe it works.

- Cut out sugar, white flour, white bread.

- I really believe in wheatgrass. It's becoming more available now. It doesn't taste good, but it does wonders for your immune system.

- Sea veggies: these are a blend of natural sea minerals that give huge doses of natural antioxidants.

- Work on your lymphatic system – rebounding is good for that.

- Avoid scans if you can, including mammograms. There are alternatives. I don't believe in PET scans or MRIs – too much damage can be done to the body through these massive doses of radiation.

- Regular doses of Vitamin D – prevents 77% of all cancer.

- Vitamin C drips, or at least take Vitamin C.

- Glutathione – an antioxidant supplement.

- Do not ever consume artificial sweeteners.

- Watch what you eat and drink – eat organic as much as possible, and keep your diet as alkaline as you can.

- Drink alkaline water – and lots of it!

- Do your blood work; keep an eye on any changes.

- Prescribe yourself massive and frequent doses of laughter (I used to watch Faulty Towers every night).

- You cannot stay in a fear mode and you cannot go inside yourself. Keep positive people around you.

- Do not give in to self-pity or rage. It is a fact that five minutes of rage will deplete your immune system for four or more hours. Why bother with those five minutes? They will achieve nothing.

- Take one day at a time. AA gave me the tools to do that. You don't have to think about tomorrow. Just focus on today.

- Think of your body like a fish tank. When it gets dirty, you clean it out. Our bodies are amazing. Our cells are always changing. If you give it what it needs to repair, it will repair itself.

- I read religiously; I read everything I could. I still do. There are several books which I have quoted from in this book and which I highly recommend. I have read them many times over, refer to them often and still use them on an almost daily basis.

And you must let go of resentment. The following quote says it perfectly.

LETTING GO
Author unknown

To let go doesn't mean to stop caring;

It means I can't do it for someone else.

To let go is not to cut myself off...

It's the realization that I can't control another...

To let go is not to enable,

but to allow learning from natural consequences.

To let go is to admit powerlessness,

which means the outcome is not in my hands.

To let go is not to try and change or blame another,

I can only change myself.

To let go is not to care for, but to care about.

To let go is not to fix, but to be supportive.

To let go is not to judge,

but to allow another to be a human being.

To let go is not to be in the middle arranging all the outcomes,

but to allow others to affect their own outcomes.

To let go is not to be protective,

It is to permit another to face reality.

To let go is not to deny, but to accept.

To let go is not to nag, scold, or argue,

but to search out my own shortcomings and correct them.

To let go is not to adjust everything to my desires,

but to take each day as it comes and cherish the moment.

To let go is not to criticize and regulate anyone,

but to try to become what I dream I can be.

To let go is not to regret the past,

but to grow and live for the future.

To let go is to fear less and love more.

In *"A Deep Breath of Life,"* published by Hay House, Alan Cohen says:

Health is our natural state, and it is within our ability to maintain good health at all times. Any notion to the contrary is a limited belief system and must be discarded without hesitation. The length and quality of your life is in your hands, and no external force has power over your vitality.

The first prescription, quiet, is essential to well-being. How can you hear the voice of God if you are preoccupied with the outer world? Each day, take time to be with yourself. Meditate, walk in the woods, or lock yourself in the bathroom. God lives not on a distant cloud, but within your heart. Spirit is not playing a hide-and-seek game. To the contrary, God is utterly desirous of being known and enjoyed. If you feel distant from God, who moved? Go to the quiet inner temple regularly, and all outer activity will be more peaceful.

Joy is as vital to good health as air. Every enlightened being I know is filled with happiness and laughter. Do not fall prey to images of God as a sombre, mournful entity. God is not a mean old man; She is a joyful child. You do not need to analyse and process every thought and experience; go out and play, laugh, get silly, and cast fear to the wind. You will find truth more quickly through delight than gravity.

Diet is extremely important. Our bodies were constructed to function at a high level of efficiency, flexibility and well-being. To keep the body healthy, we must feed it in harmony with nature. Eat fresh, live, whole, pure foods, free of artificial ingredients or preservatives. Avoid sugar, fat, salt and processed food. Make your meals a sacrament; take time to be with your food, thank God for

it, and digest it. Give your body love in the form of quality nour-
ishment, and it will respond with robust health.

"I pray to be fully healthy and manifest the well-being I deserve. I
am healthy, whole, vital and happy as I live in harmony with my
natural spirit."

This story from Alan Cohen's book also struck a chord with me.

Is That So?

That that is, is. That that is not, is not. Is that it? It is.

—Anonymous.

When a young Japanese woman became pregnant by a sailor,
she did not want the responsibility of raising the child, and named
a local monk as the father. The woman's father angrily took the
child to the gate of the monastery where the monk lived and in-
formed him, "My daughter has told me you are the father of this
child; now you must raise him."

The monk thought for a moment and answered, "Is that so?" He
took the child and cared for him as if he were his own son

Seven years later on her deathbed, the boy's mother confessed
that the child was not the monk's. Her father returned to the
monastery and humbly apologised to the monk. "My daughter has
admitted her dishonesty. I will take the child back now."

Again the monk thought for a moment, and answered, "Is that
so?"

Then he let the child go.

True mastery lies in flowing with the events of life. We are em-
powered when we assume that everything comes from God and
goes back to God. Nothing in form lasts forever, and when we can
accept change, we are free. All pain is borne of resistance. An atti-

tude of nonresistance liberates tremendous energy. Pain arises when we fight against what is happening, and peace comes when we accept what is.

What in your life are you resisting? How much peace could you gain by letting what is, be? Practice the art of allowing, and you will come close to heaven as you discover the hand of God behind everything.

Help me trust the flow of life. Show me how to accept what is, with love and appreciation.

Divine order is operating here and now.

Also, Alan Cohen writes in "*A Deep Breath of Life*":

"*Everyone is about as happy as they make up their mind to be*"

—Abraham Lincoln

The Choice for Happiness

Connie's mother-in-law was a very unhappy person. Among her many complaints, she griped that she hadn't been on a vacation in years. So Connie and her husband decided to give Mrs Fraser a luxurious Caribbean cruise. "Perhaps this will give her a lift and let her know that she is loved!" the couple hoped. After Mrs Fraser received the notice of the gift in the mail, the couple was surprised to receive a phone call from her turning down their offer. The present did not include a flight to Miami, where the cruise originated, and Mrs Fraser did not want to have to pay the fare from South Carolina.

If someone is intent on being unhappy, you cannot make them happy. A negative mind will seize on any excuse to find fault; it will find the 1/50th of the glass that is empty, overlooking the other 49 parts.

It is not within your power to choose happiness for another person, nor is it your right or purpose. If you could, you would violate their free will; perhaps they choose this situation to help them reconsider how they are living, and ultimately choose a more rewarding path. You cannot afford to make your happiness dependant on another's. You can love, bless, nurture, suggest, support, give and honour, but in the long run the only way the other person will be happy is if they choose to do so.

If you offer love or gifts to someone, and they are not received in the spirit of love, do not take it personally. The rejection is a statement of the person's pain, not your inadequacy. If you have tried for a long time to make certain people happy and have not succeeded, then just give love. Assume that they are where they need to be for a reason, and someday they will make another choice. In the meantime, be happy yourself.

I believe in mantras, quotes and prayers. Every morning, I would say this prayer:

"A New Day," by Marriane Williamson

Dear God

Thank you for this new day, its beauty and its light

Thank you for my chance to begin again

Free me from the limitations of yesterday

Today may I be reborn

May I become more fully a reflection of Your radiance

Give me strength and compassion and courage and wisdom

Show me the light in myself and others

May I recognise the good that is available everywhere

May I be, this day, an instrument of love and healing

Lead me into gentle pastures

Give me deep peace that I might serve You most deeply

Amen.

Every night I would say this:

"Evening Prayers," by Marianne Williamson

Dear God

Thank You for this day.

Thank You for my safety and the safety of my loved ones.

As I enter sleep, may these hours give me peace,

May they bring healing to my mind and body.

While I sleep, dear Lord, please bless the world.

Where there is pain, where there are people who have no place to sleep, who suffer and who die, may Your angels come unto them and minister to their lives.

Dear Lord,

Please let the light stream in.

Please use my hours of sleep.

Please prepare me, during these hours of rest, for greater service to You.

May the light that surrounds me, tomorrow shine through me.

Soften my heart.

Thank you, Lord.

Amen.

If I could leave you with some advice, it would be stolen from a medieval poem, *Regimen Sanitatis Salernitanum* – which translates to *The Salernitan Rule of Health* (commonly known as *The Flower of Medicine*, *The Lily of Medicine*) and whose author is unknown:

"Use three physicians still: first, Dr Quiet. Next, Dr Merryman, and Dr Dyet."

Those words, so simple and true, are as relevant today as when they were penned in the 12th or 13th century.

Cancer has changed my life, and that of those around me. Along the way, I have learned much, not only about the disease, but about myself. I have learned to accept the cards I have been dealt, and to make the best of them. I have cried many times, but I have also laughed.

Recently, Gary and I were at a restaurant in Palm Springs, out for dinner with my brother-in-law and his wife. Gary's brother had had prostate cancer and had a catheter fitted. I raised my glass to make a toast: "Here is to tit-less, ball-less and shit-less." My sister-in-law, who still has all her body parts, said "I feel left out!"

We laughed at the absurdity of our situation – all of us too young to be challenged by health problems, but grateful to be here anyway.

Thank you for allowing me to share my journey with you. I hope you have taken something positive and useful from it. Whatever you choose to believe, the truth remains that I have beaten cancer naturally - twice. My husband and daughter have also beaten it the same way. We are all alive and well and living in health and hope.

Whatever we have been through, are going through, or will go through in life, each of us has our own, personal journey to make. And now, I will continue with mine.

Next stop: Graceland.